Keto Bread

101 Easy and Delicious Low Carb Keto Bread Recipes for Weight Loss

Table of Contents

INTRODUCTION 1

CHAPTER 1: Baking Basics 3

    Equipment Needed 3

    Baking Skills and Techniques 5

CHAPTER 2: Keto Sweet and Savory Breads 7

    5-Ingredient Loaf Bread 7

    Dairy-Free Bread 9

    Sesame Seed Bread 12

    Coconut Bread 15

    Sweet Almond Bread 18

    Cinnamon Bread 20

    Cream Cheese Bread 22

    Blueberry Bread 25

    Savory Veggie Loaf 28

    Cheddar & Garlic Herbed Bread 31

    Zucchini Bread 33

    Mini Cheesy Loaves 35

    Basic Loaf Bread 38

    Olive & Rosemary Focaccia 40

    Cheddr Focaccia 43

CHAPTER 3: Keto Bagels 46

    Easy Cheesy Bagels 46

    Soft & Chewy Bagels 48

    Chewy Fathead Bagels 51

Rye Bagels 53

Pizza Bagels 55

Rosemary Bagels 59

Cauliflower Bagels 61

Jalapeno Bagels 64

Blueberry Cheesecake Bagels 66

Cinnamon Bagels 68

CHAPTER 4: Keto Pizza 71

Fathead Pizza Crust 71

Easy Mozzarella Crust Pizza 74

White Pizza 76

Thin Crust Pizza 79

Chicken Barbecue Pizza 81

Portobello Mushroom Personal Pizzas 83

Bell Pepper & Basil Pizza 85

Buffalo Chicken Pizza 87

Pan-Fried Pizza Margherita 90

Cinnamon Pizza 92

Fruit Dessert Pizza 95

CHAPTER 5: Keto Muffins 97

Quick-and-Easy Muffins 97

Quick-and-Easy Cinnamon Muffins 99

Quick-and-Easy Feta & Cheese Muffins 100

Quick-and-Easy Feta & Cheese Muffins 102

Cheesy Herbed Muffins 103

Egg Muffins 105

Ham & Zucchini Muffins 107

Chicken Thyme Muffins 109

Lemon Muffins 111

Blueberry & Cream Cheese Muffins 113

Chocolate Chip Muffins 115

Strawberry Muffins with Coconut Cream Glaze 118

Raspberry Muffins 120

Cranberry Muffins 122

Easy Banana Muffins 124

CHAPTER 6: Keto Crackers and Breadsticks 126

3-Ingredient Crackers 126

Rosemary & Flax Seed Crackers 128

Cheese & Basil Crackers 130

Almond & Coconut Crisps 131

Butter Crackers 134

Thyme Crackers 136

Herbed Crackers 138

Sour Cream & Chive Crackers 138

Basic Breaksticks 141

Cheesy Breaksticks 143

Italian-Style Breaksticks 144

Cinnamon Breaksticks 146

Easy Cheese & Garlic Breadsticks 147

CHAPTER 7: Keto Cookies 148

Super Easy Peanut Butter Cookies 148

Butter Cookies 150

Cream Cheese Cookies 152

Macadamia Cookies 154

Brownie Cookies 156

Basic Sugar Cookies 158

Lemon Sugar Cookies 160

Chocolate Chip Cookies 162

Walnut Cookies 164

Raspberry Cookies 166

Flourless Chocolate Chip Cookies 168

Choco Fudge Cookies 170

CHAPTER 8: Keto Bread for Breakfast, Lunch, and Dinner 172

Quick Microwaveable Bread 172

Avocado Bacon Breakfast Muffins 174

English Muffins 176

Blueberry Bread Loaf 178

Broccoli & Cheddar Breakfast Bread 180

Cloud Bread 182

Easy French Toast 184

Sandwich Bread 186

Almond Flour Loaf 188

Spinach and Feta Bread 190

Psyllium Husk & Coconut Flour Loaf 192

Flatbread 194

Buttery Garlic Bread 196

Cheese & Bacon Bread 199

Dinner Rolls 202

Irish Soda Bread 205

Microwaveable Hamburger Bun 207

Naan Bread 208

Pumpkin Bread Loaf 209

Pork Rind Bread 213

Flaxseed Tortilla Wraps 215

Basic Biscuits 217

Cheesy Garlic Biscuits 219

Yogurt Herbed Biscuits 221

Basic Almond Biscotti 223

Caramel & Chocolate Biscotti 225

CONCLUSION *228*

INTRODUCTION

This book contains 101 easy and delicious keto bread recipes to fill you up during your ketogenic diet.

If you think that you'd need to give up bread forever when going through a ketogenic diet, think again. You can still enjoy a scrumptious meal without sacrificing bread by making the recipes in this book.

You'll find tons of recipes from pizzas to loaf breads to muffins, which are all low in carbohydrates. The key is to use ingredients that are low in carbs and high in fat.

After making these recipes, you don't need to go through another day without your favorite breads. The Recipe instructions are so easy and simple that even a beginner can do. These breads are perfect for breakfast, lunch, dinner, and snack time.

You'll also find the nutritional numbers for each recipe, so you can keep track of your macros every day. But take note that numbers may vary depending on the brand of the ingredients used.

For a first-time keto bread baker, you may need to experiment on the best brands to use for the recipes. But once you've gotten used to it, baking your favorite keto breads will be easier.

You don't have to settle for a breadless meal when you can make perfect bread recipes that'll fit your diet. Browse through 101 recipes that you can make every day.

Thanks for downloading this book, I hope you enjoy it!

CHAPTER 1

Baking Basics

If you haven't baked anything before, then you'll need to have the basic equipment and learn techniques so you can bake all the yummy recipes in this book.

Baking is not as difficult as you think. If you follow the directions as well as specific measurements of the ingredients then it's impossible to fail.

Equipment Needed

Oven

You'd need a functioning oven to bake your bread. Some recipes may only require frying with a pan, but most bread recipes would need an oven. In the book, you'll find the temperature setting for each recipe. But, these are for conventional ovens. If you're using a convection oven, you may need to research on the equivalent temperature for it.

Baking sheets and tins

You'll also need baking sheets and tins where you'll place your dough or batter to bake the bread. There's a wide selection of non-stick baking sheets and tins you can buy that will help you remove your bread easier after baking. You'd need a few baking sheets, loaf tins, and muffins tins.

Parchment paper

Parchment paper is a type of paper that won't burn even in high temperatures. These are used to line the baking sheets and tins so the bread won't stick. Even though you're using non-stick sheets and tins, it's best to use parchment paper. You'll also need these to easily roll out sticky dough and batter easily.

Mixing bowls

You'll need lots of mixing bowls of different sizes. You may need large ones for large batches of bread. Small ones are useful for mixing small amounts of wet and dry mixtures.

Measuring cups and spoons

Baking is all about precise measurements to get the best outcome. You'll need accurate measuring tools to measure out the ingredients for each bread recipe.

Mixing tools

Having electric stand and hand mixers will make mixing such an ease. Making large recipes will be tiring if you'll use a whisk or spatula and mix by hand. If you don't have any electric mixers, you can still follow the recipes and mix by hand. But, you have to be ready for an arm workout. Spatulas would also be needed when you have to fold your ingredients together.

Rolling pin

A rolling pin will help you roll out the dough when you need to flatten it. This'll be useful for many recipes in this book.

Baking Skills and Techniques

Mixing

Mixing the ingredients is easier when using an electric mixer. But, mixing by hand is also possible. It may just take more time and energy. Don't be discouraged when you find that your mixture doesn't seem to come together, it'll get better once you start kneading.

Kneading

After mixing all the bread ingredients, knead it to make the dough elastic and smooth. Some of the bread recipes in this book won't require kneading because of their fluid-like consistency. It would take

5-10 minutes depending on the recipe. After kneading, your dough should hold its shape together.

Toothpick Test

The toothpick test would need a toothpick, knife, or skewer poked into the bread to know if it's done. If the toothpick comes out clean, the bread is done. If some of the bread sticks to the toothpick, it means that it needs more cooking.

Shaping the dough

You also need to learn how to shape the dough depending on the type of bread you're making. You may need bread-shaping tools to shape the dough correctly.

CHAPTER 2

Keto Sweet and Savory Breads

5-Ingredient Loaf Bread

Yields: 1 loaf (18 pieces ½" slices)

Nutrition Facts: Amount per serving (½" slice)

- ➢ Carbohydrates – 3g
- ➢ Protein – 4g
- ➢ Total Fat – 7g
- ➢ Calories – 82

Ingredients:

a. 1 cup blanched almond flour

b. ¼ cup coconut flour

c. 2 tsp. baking powder, gluten-free

d. ¼ tsp. sea salt

e. 1/3 cup butter, melted

f. 12 large egg whites

Directions:

1. Preheat your oven to 325° F (165° C). Then, line a 4.5x8.5-inch loaf pan with parchment paper.
2. Mix the dry ingredients until well-combined.
3. Add in the butter and combine until crumbly.
4. In a large bowl, beat the egg whites until stiff peaks form. Use cream of tartar for easy whipping if preferred.
5. Fold in the egg white mixture to the flour mixture gently.
6. Then transfer the flour+egg white mixture to the bowl with the remaining egg whites.
7. Fold the mixture gently and keep as much fluffiness as possible.
8. Transfer the mixture to your loaf pan and smoothen.
9. Bake for 40 minutes or until golden brown.
10. Using aluminum foil, tent the top of the loaf pan. Bake for 30-45 minutes more until the top is firm and it doesn't make any squishy sounds when you press it.
11. Remove the bread from the oven. Cool it before removing from the loaf pan. Slice into ½-inch pieces.

Dairy-Free Bread

Yields: 4 buns

Nutrition Facts: Amount per serving (1 bun)

- Carbohydrates – 7.5g
- Protein – 6.5g
- Total Fat – 13.4g
- Calories – 170

Ingredients:

a. 2 oz. macadamia butter
b. 1 oz. coconut flour, sifted
c. ½ tbsp. psyllium husk powder
d. ½ tsp. baking powder
e. ½ tsp. Erythritol sweetener
f. ¼ tsp. salt
g. 2 large eggs + 1 large egg white

Directions:

1. Preheat your oven to 350° F (180° C.) Line a baking sheet with parchment paper.
2. Mix all the dry ingredients except the psyllium husk powder in a bowl.

3. In a separate bowl, beat the eggs. Add the macadamia butter and mix until well-combined.
4. Mix the dry and wet mixtures together. Then, add in the psyllium husk powder. If the mixture seems a bit watery, add a tablespoon of coconut flour.
5. Divide the dough into 4 and form into disks. Place the dough disks onto the baking sheet.
6. Bake for 30 minutes or until they pass the toothpick test. Let them cool before serving.

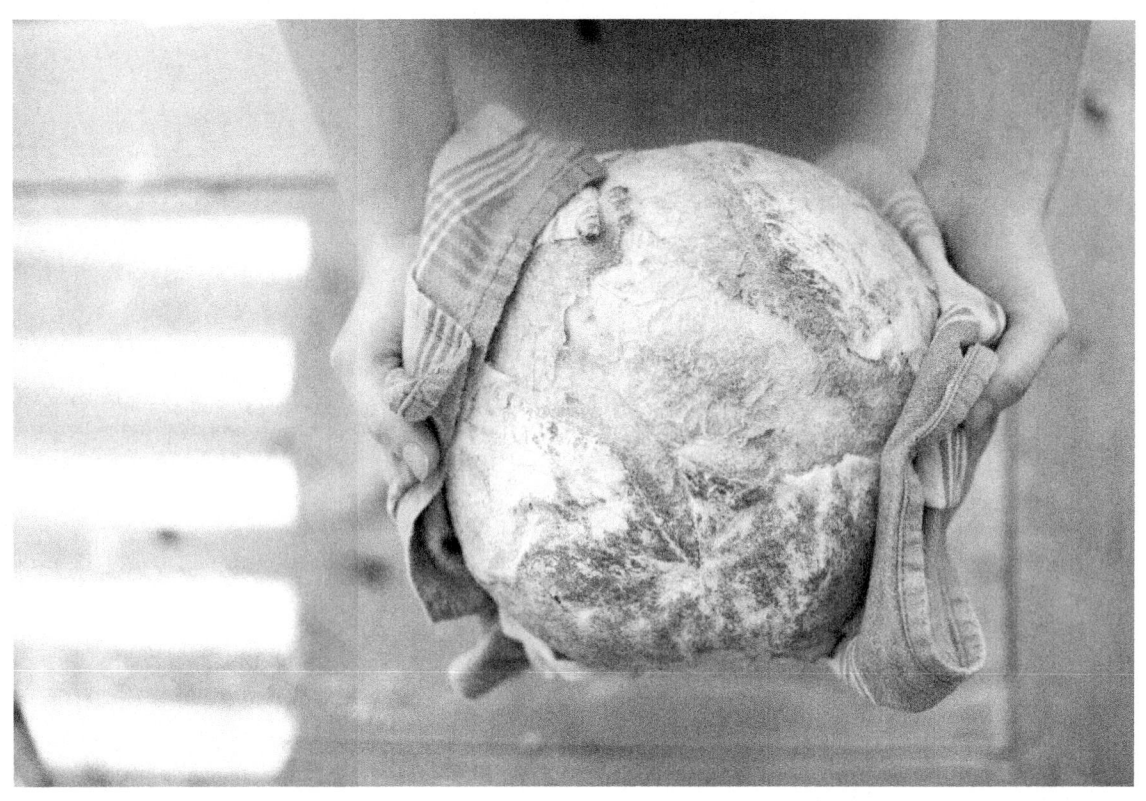

Sesame Seed Bread

Yields: 1 loaf (16 slices)

Nutrition Facts: Amount per serving (2 slices)

- ➢ Carbohydrates – 10g
- ➢ Protein – 17g
- ➢ Total Fat – 30g
- ➢ Calories – 368

Ingredients:

- a. 2 cups sesame seed flour
- b. ½ cup unsalted butter, melted
- c. 1 tsp. baking powder
- d. ½ tsp. salt
- e. 7 large eggs, yolks and whites separated

Directions:

1. Preheat the oven to 355° F (180° C). Use parchment paper to line a loaf tin.
2. Beat the egg whites until opaque and fluffy.
3. In another bowl, mix the egg yolks. Add in the rest of the ingredients.

4. Then, fold in the egg yolk mixture into the egg whites until well-combined.
5. Transfer the mixture to the loaf tin. Bake for 45 minutes or until it passes the toothpick test.
6. Remove and bread for the loaf tin and slice into 16 pieces.

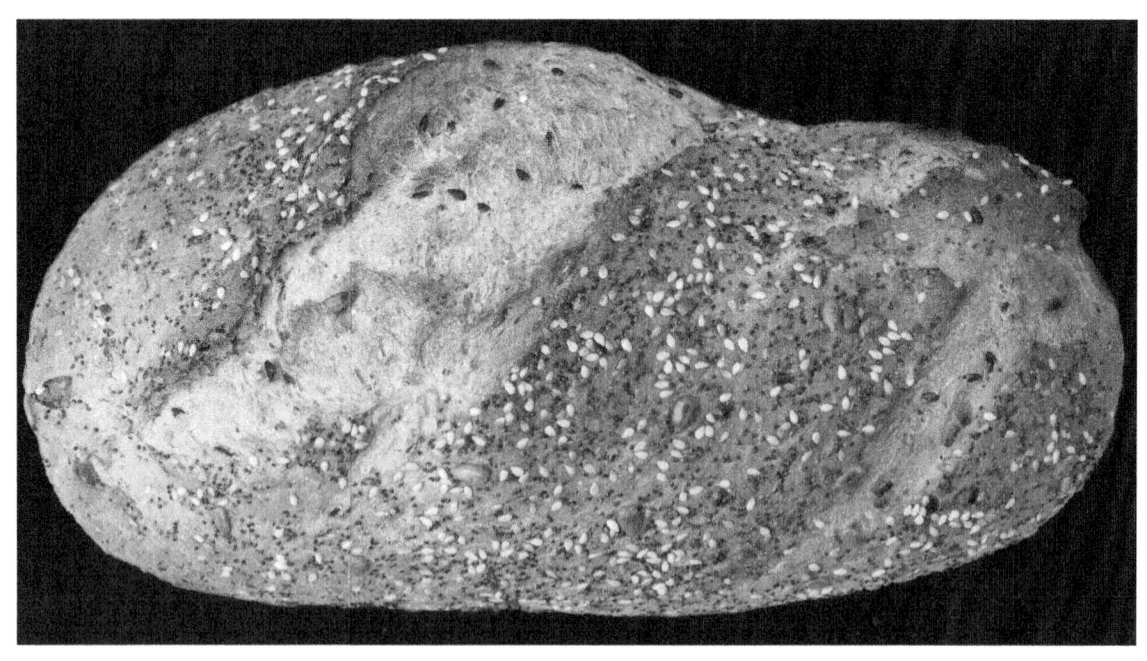

Coconut Bread

Yields: 1 loaf (16 slices)

Nutrition Facts: Amount per serving (2 slices)

- Carbohydrates – 3.5g
- Protein – 6g
- Total Fat – 17g
- Calories – 191

Ingredients:

a. ½ cup coconut flour

b. ½ cup butter

c. ½ tsp. xanthan gum

d. ¼ tsp. salt.

e. ¼ tsp. baking powder, aluminum-free

f. 7 large eggs

Directions:

1. Preheat your oven to 355° F (180° C.) Prepare a 5x8.5-inch loaf tin lined with parchment paper.
2. Beat the eggs well before adding the rest of the ingredients. Mix until you get a thick mixture.
3. Pour the mixture into the loaf tin and smoothen the top.

4. Bake for about 50 minutes or do the toothpick test using a skewer. When it comes out clean, it's done.
5. Remove from the tin and cut into 16 slices

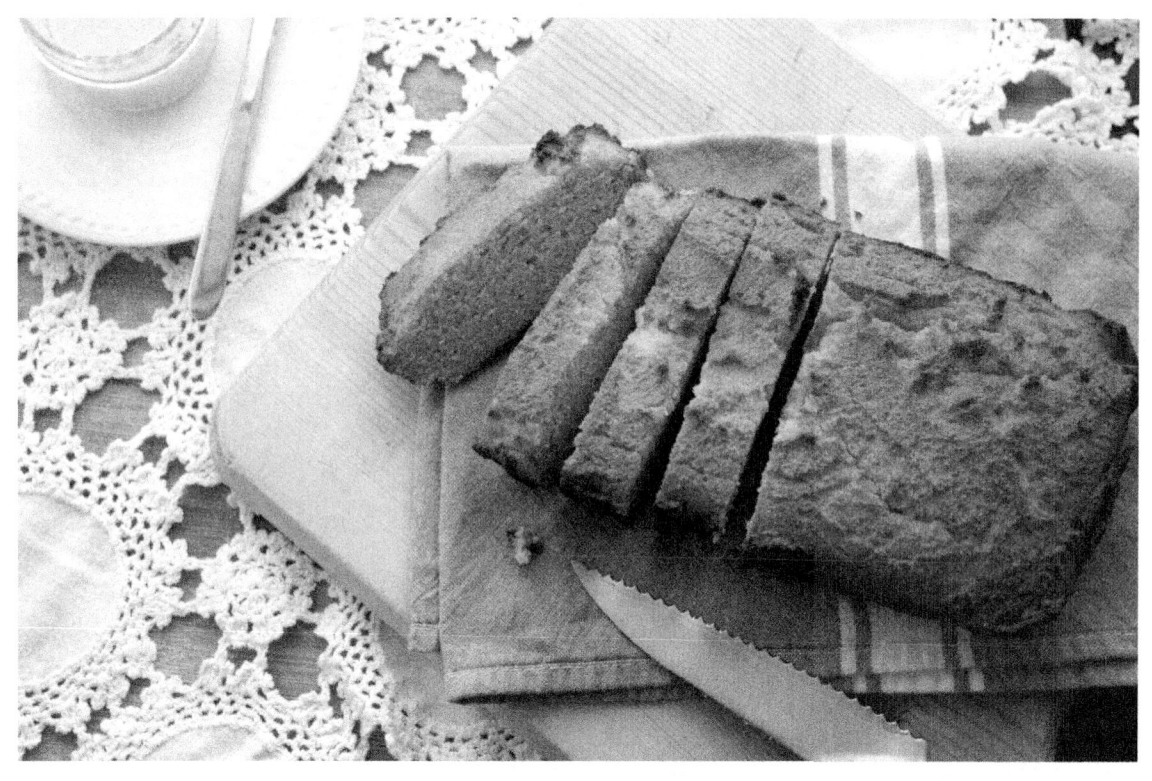

Sweet Almond Bread

Yields: 1 loaf (14 slices)

Nutrition Facts: Amount per serving (1 slice)

- ➢ Carbohydrates – 4.5g
- ➢ Protein – 5.2g
- ➢ Total Fat – 19.8g
- ➢ Calories – 206

Ingredients:

a. 2 ¼ cups almond flour
b. ½ cup Stevia sweetener
c. ½ cup butter
d. ½ cup heavy cream
e. 2 tbsp. flaxseed, ground
f. 1 tsp. baking powder
g. ½ tsp. xanthan gum
h. ¼ tsp. ginger powder
i. ¼ tsp. star anise, ground
j. 2 eggs

Directions:

1. Preheat the oven to 350° F (175° C.) Line a loaf tin with parchment paper.
2. In a pot, melt the butter over medium heat. Then, add in the heavy cream and Stevia. Stir until the sugar dissolves.
3. Remove from the heat and let it cool to almost room temperature.
4. Mix all the remaining dry ingredients in a large bowl.
5. Add the butter mixture and 2 eggs to the dry ingredients. Mix everything together.
6. Pour the batter into the loaf tin. Bake for 45 minutes. Cover the top with parchment paper if it's starting to brown quickly. Let it cool before slicing into 14.

Cinnamon Bread

Yields: 1 loaf (10 slices)

Nutrition Facts: Amount per serving (1 slice)

- ➢ Carbohydrates – 2.5g
- ➢ Protein – 5.8g
- ➢ Total Fat – 15.7g
- ➢ Calories – 172

Ingredients:

a. 3 oz. cream cheese, softened
b. 1 cup almond flour
c. ¼ cup Erythritol sweetener
d. 4 tbsp. butter (separate 2 tbsp. melted and 2 tbsp. softened)
e. 1 ½ tsp cinnamon (divided into ½ tsp. and 1 tsp.
f. 1 tsp. vanilla
g. 1 tsp. baking powder
h. ¼ tsp. cream of tartar
i. 12 drops of liquid Stevia
j. 4 eggs, yolk and whites separated

Directions:

1. Preheat your oven to 350° F (175° C). Grease a 9x5-inch loaf tin.
2. Beat the egg whites with the cream of tartar until soft peaks form.
3. In another bowl, mix the egg yolks, vanilla, Stevia, cream cheese, and softened butter until well-combined.
4. Add ½ tsp. cinnamon, flour, and baking powder to the egg yolk mixture and mix well.
5. Mix the remaining cinnamon, Erythritol and melted butter in another bowl. Set it aside.
6. Combine the egg whites and egg yolk mixture. Fold them together gently.
7. Take half of the egg mixture and place in the loaf tin. Evenly spread the butter and cinnamon mixture on top.
8. Pour in the remaining egg mixture making and spread out evenly.
9. Use a butter knife to create swirls in the batter. But, avoid mixing too much.
10. Bake for 40 minutes or until golden brown. Remove from the loaf tin, slice into 10 pieces, and serve.

Cream Cheese Bread

Yields: 1 loaf (12 slices)

Nutrition Facts: Amount per serving (1 slice)

- Carbohydrates – 2.2g
- Protein – 5.8g
- Total Fat – 19.4g
- Calories – 204

Ingredients:

a. 8 oz. full-fat cream cheese, softened
b. 1 ½ cups coconut flour
c. ½ cup unsalted butter, softened
d. ½ cup full-fat sour cream
e. 2 tbsp. sesame seeds
f. 1 tbsp. Stevia sweetener
g. 4 tsp. baking powder
h. 1 tsp. sea salt
i. 8 eggs, room temperature

Directions:

1. Grease a 5x10-inch loaf tin with butter and preheat the oven to 350° F (175° C).

2. Combine the dry ingredients except the sesame seeds in a bowl. Set aside.
3. Beat the butter and cream cheese together. Then, add in the eggs one at a time while continuing to mix.
4. Add the dry mixture to the wet mixture slowly and continue stirring.
5. Next, fold in the sour cream to the combined mixture.
6. Transfer the batter to the loaf tin. Bake for about an hour or more if you think that it needs more cooking time.
7. Remove from the loaf tin and slice it into 12 pieces before serving.

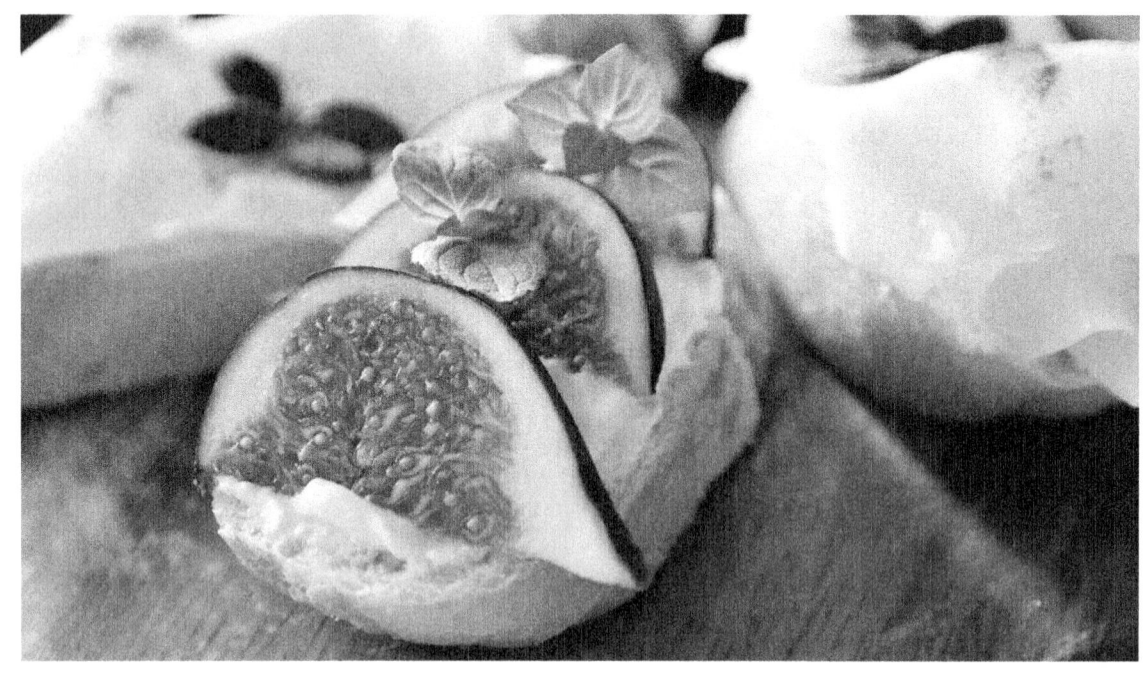

Blueberry Bread

Yields: 1 loaf (12 slices)

Nutrition Facts: Amount per serving (1 slice)

- ➤ Carbohydrates –4g
- ➤ Protein – 3g
- ➤ Total Fat – 13g
- ➤ Calories – 155

Ingredients: (Bread)

a. ¾ cup blueberries, fresh
b. 2/3 cup Monkfruit sweetener (can be decreased if you want a less sweet bread)
c. 10 tbsp. coconut flour
d. 9 tbsp. butter, melted
e. 2 tbsp. sour cream
f. 2 tbsp. heavy whipping cream
g. 1 ½ tsp. vanilla
h. 1 ½ tsp. baking powder
i. ½ tsp. salt
j. ½ tsp. cinnamon
k. 6 eggs

(Icing)

 a. 2 tbsp. Monkfruit sweetener

 b. 1 tbsp. heavy whipping cream

 c. 1 tsp. butter, melted

 d. ¼ tsp. lemon zest

 e. 1/8 tsp. vanilla

Directions:

1. Line a loaf tin with parchment paper and preheat the oven to 350° F (175° C).
2. Combine all the bread ingredients except the butter, coconut flour, and blueberries.
3. Mix in the butter. And finally, mix in the coconut flour.
4. Layer a small amount of batter in the loaf tin. Then, top with blueberries. Repeat the process until all the blueberries and batter are in the tin. This will evenly distribute the blueberries in your bread.
5. Bake for 65 minutes or do the toothpick test using a knife. The bread is done if the knife comes out clean.
6. Let it cool for about 5 minutes. During this time, combine all the icing ingredients. Whisk until you get a smooth mixture.

7. Cut the bread into 12 slices and drizzle the icing on top before serving.

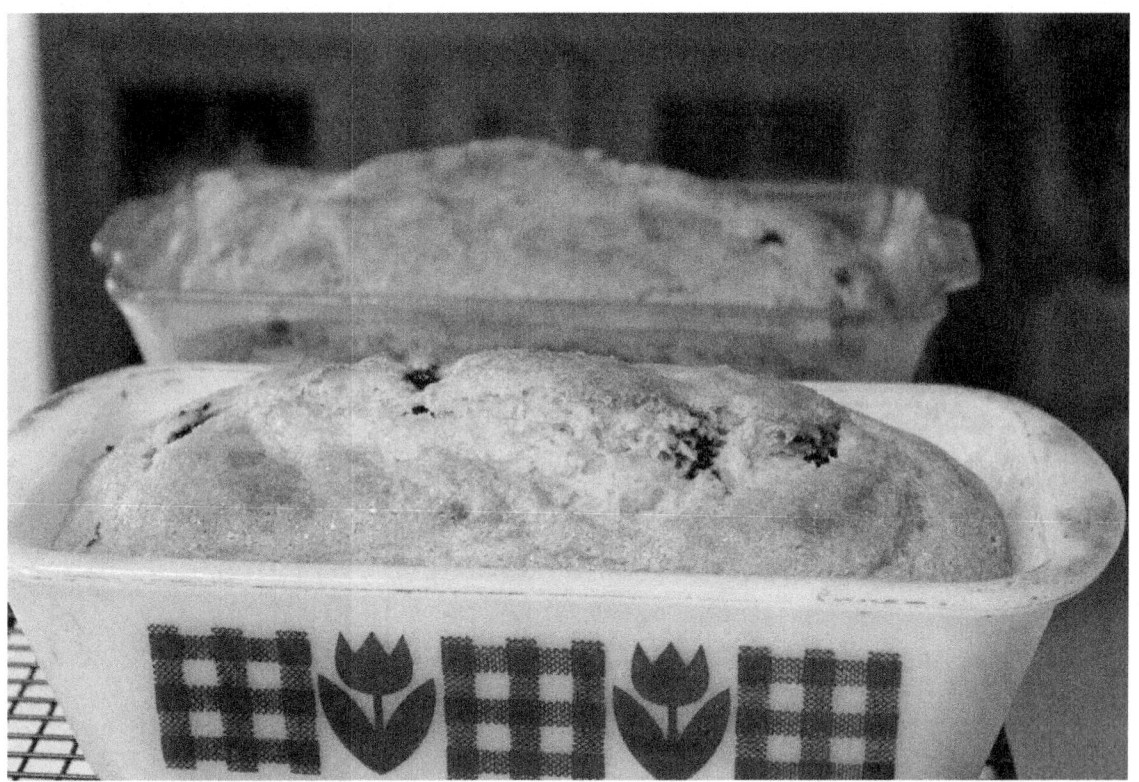

Savory Veggie Loaf

Yields: 1 loaf (12 slices)

Nutrition Facts: Amount per serving (1 slice)

- ➢ Carbohydrates – 6.8g
- ➢ Protein – 6.7g
- ➢ Total Fat – 14.5g
- ➢ Calories – 175

Ingredients:

a. 1 cup almond flour
b. ½ cup mixed pumpkin, sunflower, flaxseeds, sesame or other seeds you prefer + 2 tbsp. mixed seeds for garnishing
c. 1/3 cup coconut flour
d. ¼ cup coconut oil or ghee
e. 2 tbsp. psyllium husk powder
f. 1 tbsp. paprika, smoked
g. 2 tsp. cumin, ground
h. 2 tsp. pink Himalayan salt
i. 2 tsp. baking powder
j. 1 large zucchini, grated (320g)
k. 1 small carrot, grated (50g)
l. 1 cup pumpkin, grated (115g)

m. 4 large eggs

Directions:

1. Preheat the oven to 340° F (170° C). Line a loaf tin with parchment paper.
2. In a large bowl, mix the almond and coconut flours, salt, spices, baking powder, mixed seeds, and psyllium husk powder until they're well-combined.
3. In a separate bowl, combine the vegetables, eggs, and coconut oil (or ghee).
4. Then, add the dry ingredient mixture to the vegetable mixture and mix well.
5. Transfer the mixture to the loaf tin and lightly press down. Sprinkle the top with the mixed seed garnish.
6. Bake for 55- 70 minutes or do the toothpick test with a skewer until it pulls out clean.
7. Allow the bread to cool for about 30 minutes before moving to a cooling rack.
8. Slice into 12 pieces before serving. You can also store it in the fridge up to 5 days or in the freezer for about 3 months in an airtight container.

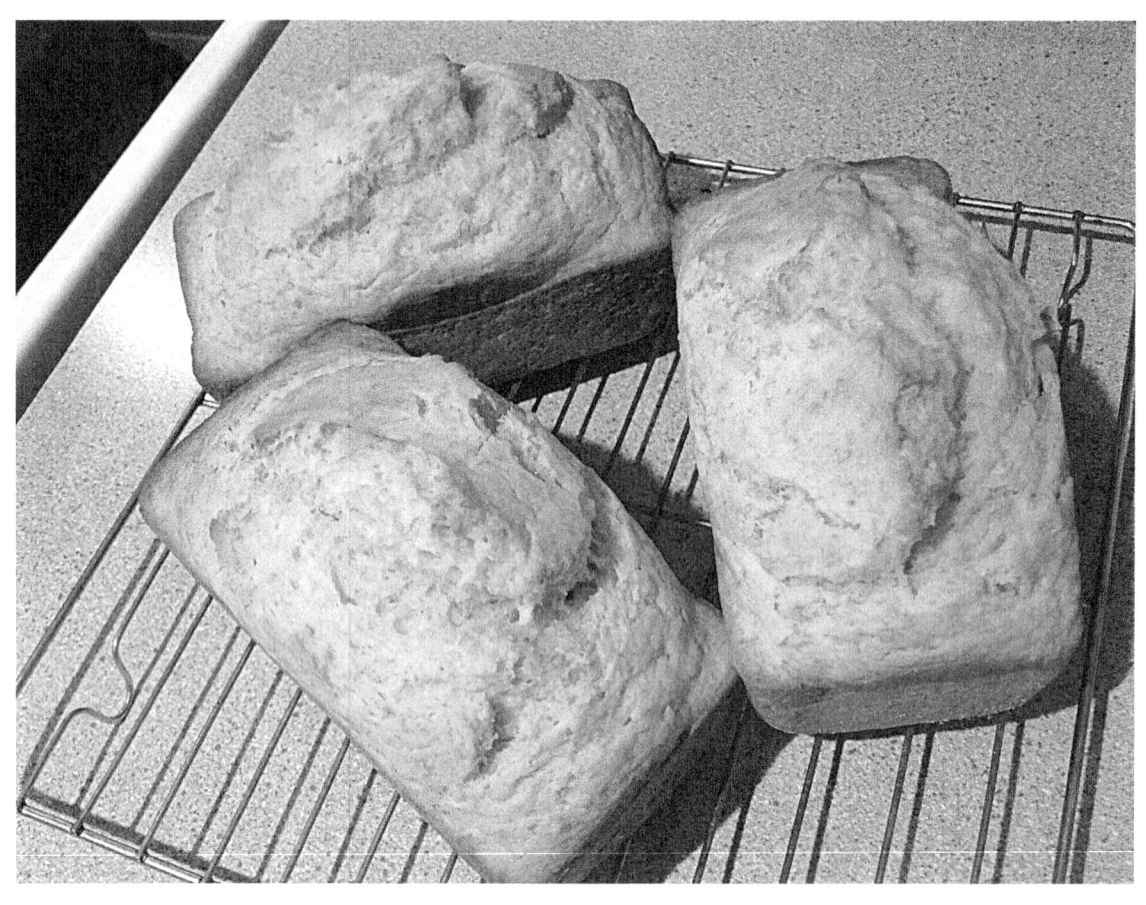

Cheddar & Garlic Herbed Bread

Yields: 1 loaf (16 slices)

Nutrition Facts: Amount per serving (1 slice)

- ➢ Carbohydrates – 4g
- ➢ Protein – 7g
- ➢ Total Fat – 10.5g
- ➢ Calories – 201

Ingredients:

a. 2 cups almond flour
b. 1 ½ cups cheddar cheese, grated (separate 1 cup and ½ cup)
c. ½ cup butter, softened
d. 2 tbsp. garlic powder
e. 1 tbsp. parsley flakes
f. ½ tbsp. oregano
g. 1 tsp. baking powder
h. ½ tsp. salt
i. ½ tsp. xanthan gum
j. 6 eggs

Directions:

1. Line a loaf tin with parchment paper and preheat your oven to 355° F (180° C).
2. Beat the eggs in a mixing bowl until frothy.
3. Add the butter to the eggs and mix well.
4. Then, mix in the baking powder. Add in the almond flour in small batches while mixing. Blend well until you get a thick mixture.
5. Next, add the 1 cup cheddar, garlic powder, parsley, and oregano and mix well.
6. Pour the batter into the loaf tin and top with the remaining cheese.
7. Bake for 45 minutes or check if the bread is done using the toothpick test.
8. Cool the bread and cut into 16 slices before serving.

Zucchini Bread

Yields: 1 loaf (12 slices)

Nutrition Facts: Amount per serving (1 slice)

- Carbohydrates – 8g
- Protein – 7g
- Total Fat – 16g
- Calories – 202

Ingredients:

a. 1 cup almond flour
b. ¾ cup + 1 tbsp. coconut flour
c. 2/3 cup zucchini, grated
d. ½ cup Monkfruit or other sugar substitute
e. 1/3 cup butter, melted
f. ¼ cup pecans, chopped
g. 3 tbsp. sour cream
h. 1 ½ tsp. baking powder
i. 1 tsp. baking soda
j. 1 tsp. cinnamon
k. 1 tsp. vanilla extract

l. ½ tsp salt

m. 8 eggs

Directions:

1. Grease a 9-inch loaf tin and line with parchment paper. Preheat your oven to 350° F (175° C).
2. Beat the eggs until you get a light and foamy texture. The volume should be tripled.
3. Add the other ingredients to the eggs except for the butter, sour cream, and vanilla extract. Mix everything until they're well-combined.
4. Mix in the remaining ingredients.
5. Transfer the batter to the loaf tin and smoothen the top. Evenly scatter the pecans on top of the batter.
6. Bake for 35 minutes up to an hour. Halfway through baking, cover the top with parchment paper to avoid the top from browning quickly. Do the toothpick test to check if the bread is done.
7. Let it cool before removing from the loaf tin. Slice into 12 pieces and serve. Store the bread in the fridge or freezer wrapped in parchment paper.

Mini Cheesy Loaves

Yields: 12 mini loaves

Nutrition Facts: Amount per serving (1 mini loaf)

- Carbohydrates – 2.8g
- Protein – 6.4g
- Total Fat – 13.8g
- Calories – 170

Ingredients:

a. 1 cup cheddar cheese, grated
b. ½ cup butter, softened
c. ½ cup coconut flour
d. ½ spring onion, finely chopped
e. 1 tsp. baking powder
f. A pinch of salt and pepper
g. A pinch of chili
h. 1 stick of pepperoni, sliced thinly
i. 2 tbsp. pumpkin seeds
j. 8 eggs

Directions:

1. Preheat your oven to 350° F (180° C). Grease a 6-piece mini loaf tin (or a muffin tin).
2. Combine the butter, coconut flour, salt, pepper, baking powder, and chili in a mixing bowl until smooth.
3. Add the eggs one at a time while stirring.
4. Add the spring onions and grated cheese. Spare some cheese to put on top of the loaves.
5. Fill the loaf tin and top the loaves with pepperoni, cheese, and pumpkin seeds.
6. Bake for 15 minutes or until they become golden brown and serve.

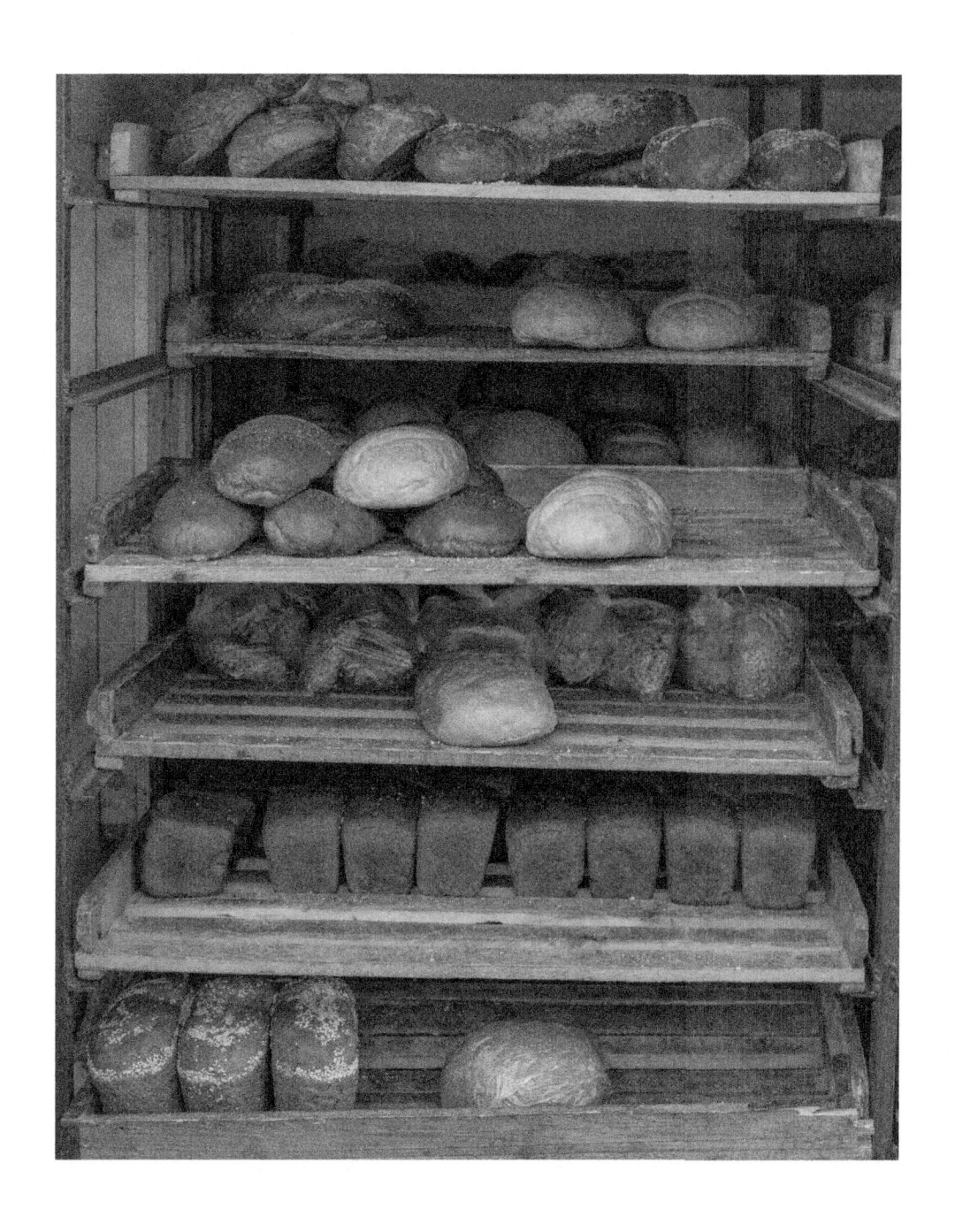

Basic Loaf Bread

Yields: 1 loaf (10 slices)

Nutrition Facts: Amount per serving (1 slice)

- Carbohydrates – 6g
- Protein – 7g
- Total Fat – 16g
- Calories – 189

Ingredients:

a. 1 ½ cups almond flour
b. ¼ cup flaxseed meal, ground
c. ¼ cup coconut oil
d. 2 tbsp. coconut flour
e. 1 tbsp. apple cider vinegar
f. 1 ½ tsp. baking soda
g. 1 tsp. Stevia sweetener
h. ¼ tsp. salt
i. 5 eggs

Directions:

1. Preheat your oven to 350° F (180° C). Grease an 8x4-inch loaf tin with coconut oil or butter.
2. Combine the dry ingredients and mix well.
3. Then, stir in the wet ingredients. Make sure everything's well-combined.
4. Pour the batter into the loaf tin and bake for 30 minutes.
5. Cool and slice into 10 pieces before serving.

Olive & Rosemary Focaccia

Yields: 10 pieces

Nutrition Facts: Amount per serving (1 piece)

- ➢ Carbohydrates – 5g
- ➢ Protein – 8g
- ➢ Total Fat – 26g
- ➢ Calories – 284

Ingredients:

a. 4 oz. cream cheese, softened
b. 4 oz. salted butter, softened
c. 1 ¾ cups almond flour
d. 1 tsp. baking powder
e. ½ tsp. garlic powder
f. ¼ tsp. xanthan gum
g. 3 rosemary sprigs
h. 16 kalamata olives, pitted and sliced
i. 4 eggs

Directions:

1. Preheat the oven to 375° F (190° C). Line an 8x12-inch baking sheet with parchment paper.
2. Whip the butter and cream cheese until fluffy. Then, add the eggs one at a time while continuing to whisk.
3. Add the rest of the ingredients except for the rosemary and olives. Combine well.
4. Pour the batter onto the baking sheet and smoothen. Then, top with the rosemary and olives. Make sure to distribute evenly.
5. Bake for 18-25 minutes or until it's a bit springy when touched. Slice into 10 equal portions before serving.

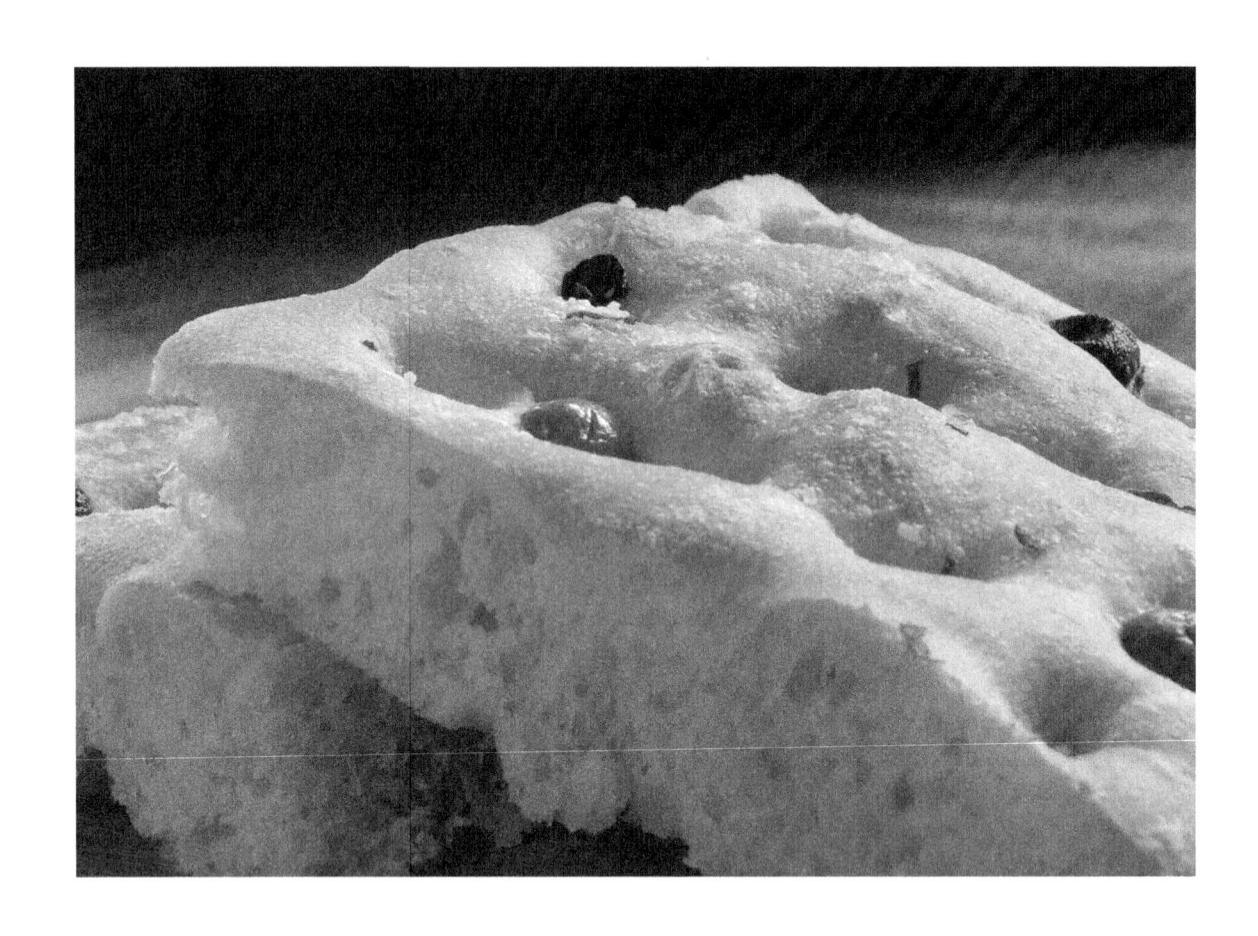

Cheddr Focaccia

Yields: 20 pieces

Nutrition Facts: Amount per serving (1 piece)

- Carbohydrates – 2g
- Protein – 6g
- Total Fat – 11g
- Calories – 131

Ingredients: (Focaccia)

a. 2 cups almond flour, finely ground
b. ¾ cup ricotta
c. ½ cup cheddar, grated
d. 3 tbsp. butter, melted
e. 1 tsp. baking soda
f. ¼ tsp. sea salt, finely ground
g. ¼ tsp. black pepper
h. 3 eggs

(Topping)

a. 1 cup cheddar, grated
b. 1 tsp. dried rosemary
c. ½ tsp. salt

Directions:

1. Preheat the oven to 375° F (190° C). Grease a 9x13-inch baking sheet coconut oil or butter.
2. Mix all the focaccia ingredients together until well-blended.
3. Then, transfer the batter onto the baking sheet and smooth out.
4. Mix the topping ingredients together in a bowl before sprinkling over the batter.
5. Bake for 25 minutes and cool before slicing into 20 equal portions.

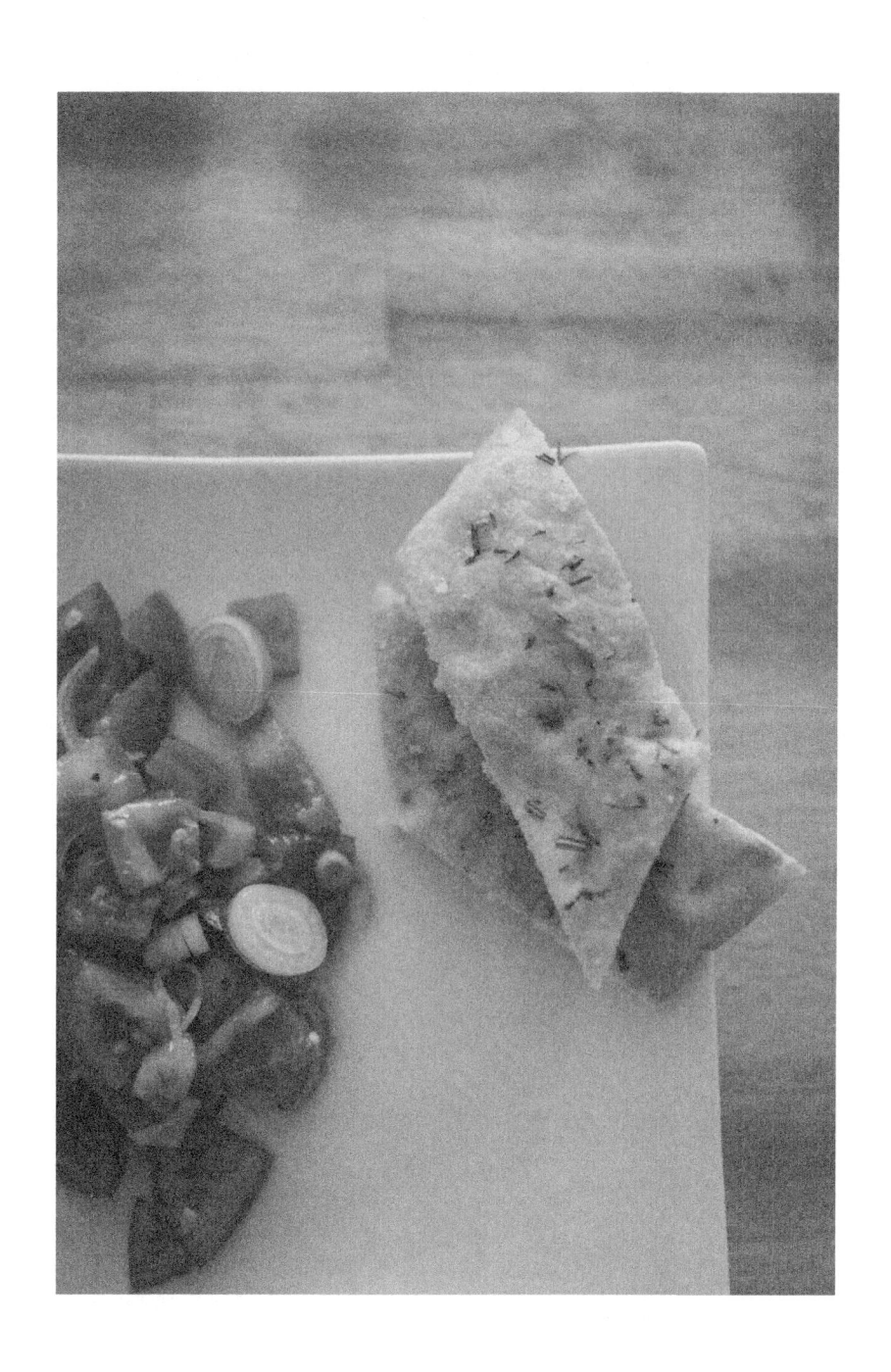

CHAPTER 3

Keto Bagels

Easy Cheesy Bagels

Yields: 6 bagels

Nutrition Facts: Amount per serving (1 bagel)

- Carbohydrates – 5g
- Protein –14g
- Total Fat – 16g
- Calories – 218

Ingredients:

a. 1 cup melty cheese (mozzarella, cheddar, or others)
b. ½ cup hard, dry cheese (parmesan, arsiago, or others)
c. 2 tbsp. everything bagel seasoning (homemade or store-bought)
d. 2 eggs

Directions:

1. Preheat the oven to 375° F (190° C). Grease a 6-piece donut pan.
2. Combine all the ingredients except the seasoning very well.
3. Separate the mixture into six parts and press into the donut pan.
4. Sprinkle the seasoning over the bagels.
5. Bake for 15 to 20 minutes. The cheese should fully melt creating a slightly brown crust.
6. Cool the bagels and serve.

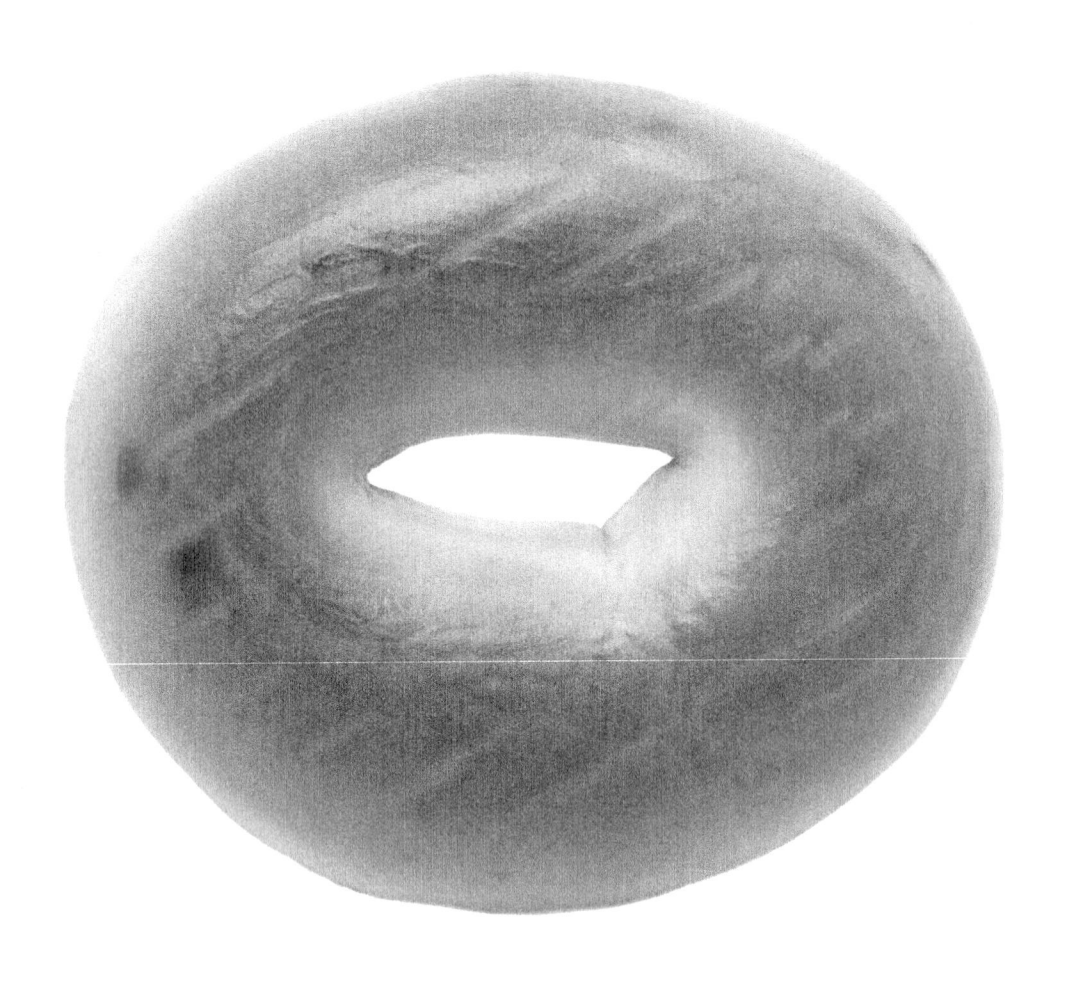

Soft & Chewy Bagels

Yields: 8 bagels

Nutrition Facts: Amount per serving (1 bagel)

- Carbohydrates – 9g
- Protein – 6g
- Total Fat – 15g
- Calories – 190

Ingredients:

a. 2 cups almond flour
b. ½ cup water, between 105° F-110° F
c. 1/3 cup psyllium husks, ground finely
d. ¼ cup whey protein isolate
e. 1 ½ tbsp. extra virgin olive oil
f. 1 tbsp. apple cider vinegar
g. 1 tbsp. active dry yeast
h. 2 ½ tsp. xanthan gum
i. 2 tsp. inulin powder
j. 2 tsp. baking powder
k. ½ to ¾ tsp. kosher salt
l. 1 egg + 2 eggs whites, left at room temperature

m. 1 egg white, beaten for egg wash

n. Everything bagel seasoning (homemade or store-bought) for topping

Directions:

1. Combine the inulin powder and yeast in a bowl. Pour in the lukewarm water, cover, and leave for 7 minutes.
2. Mix the psyllium, flour, whey protein, baking powder, xanthan gum, and salt in a separate bowl until well-combined.
3. After proofing the yeast, add in the eggs, vinegar, and olive oil. Whisk until frothy.
4. Divide the flour mixture into two. Add the flour mixture to the egg and yeast mixture 1 batch at a time while mixing.
5. Divide the dough into 8 portions and shape into bagels. Place them on a flat surface with parchment paper.
6. Cover the bagels with plastic wrap for 20-60 minutes. The longer the bagels rest, the fluffier they'll get. Preheat the oven to 350° F (180° C) while the bagels rest.
7. After resting, brush with egg wash and top with everything bagel seasoning.
8. Bake for 20-25 minutes until golden brown. But, cover the bagels with aluminum foil halfway through baking.
9. Remove the bagels from the oven and cool before serving.

Chewy Fathead Bagels

Yields: 8 bagels

Nutrition Facts: Amount per serving (1 bagel)

- ➢ Carbohydrates – 5.5g
- ➢ Protein – 12.1g
- ➢ Total Fat – 12.3g
- ➢ Calories – 190

Ingredients:

a. 12 oz. mozzarella, shredded part-skim

b. ½ cup coconut flour

c. 1 tbsp. butter, melted

d. 2 tsp. baking powder

e. ¾ tsp. xanthan gum

f. Everything bagel seasoning (store-bought or homemade) for topping

g. 2 large eggs

Directions:

1. Preheat the oven to 350° F (180° C). Prepare a large baking sheet and line with parchment paper

2. Mix the baking powder, xanthan gum, and coconut flour in a medium mixing bowl. Set aside.
3. Melt the mozzarella in a microwave. Stir every after 30 minutes until it's almost liquid.
4. Add the eggs+flour mixture to the melted mozzarella and mix until well-combined.
5. Knead the dough until completely combined. Divide the dough into 8 pieces and form into bagels.
6. Brush the tops with butter and dip into the 'everything bagel' seasoning. Place them on the baking sheet.
7. Bake for about 15 minutes or until they rise and become golden brown.
8. Let the bagels cool before serving.

Rye Bagels

Yields: 4 bagels

Nutrition Facts: Amount per serving (1 bagel)

- ➢ Carbohydrates – 11g
- ➢ Protein – 22g
- ➢ Total Fat – 18g
- ➢ Calories – 278

Ingredients:

a. 1 oz. cream cheese

b. 1 ½ cups mozzarella, shredded part-skim

c. 1 cup almond flour

d. 1 tsp. caraway seeds

e. ½ tbsp. cocoa powder

f. 1 ½ tsp. baking powder

g. 1 tsp. yacon syrup

h. 1 large egg

Directions:

1. Prepare a baking sheet and line with parchment paper. Preheat your oven to 325° F (165° C).

2. Whisk the egg in a separate bowl and set aside.

3. Mix all the ingredients except for the cheeses until well-combined.
4. Melt the cream cheese and mozzarella for 1 minute in the microwave. Take it out and stir. Microware for 30 minutes more and stir again
5. Mix in the whisked egg and flour mixture to the cheese until you form a dough.
6. Divide the dough into 4 and shape into bagels. Put them on the prepared baking sheet.
7. Bake for about 15 minutes or until them become firm and golden brown.
8. Cool the bagels and serve.

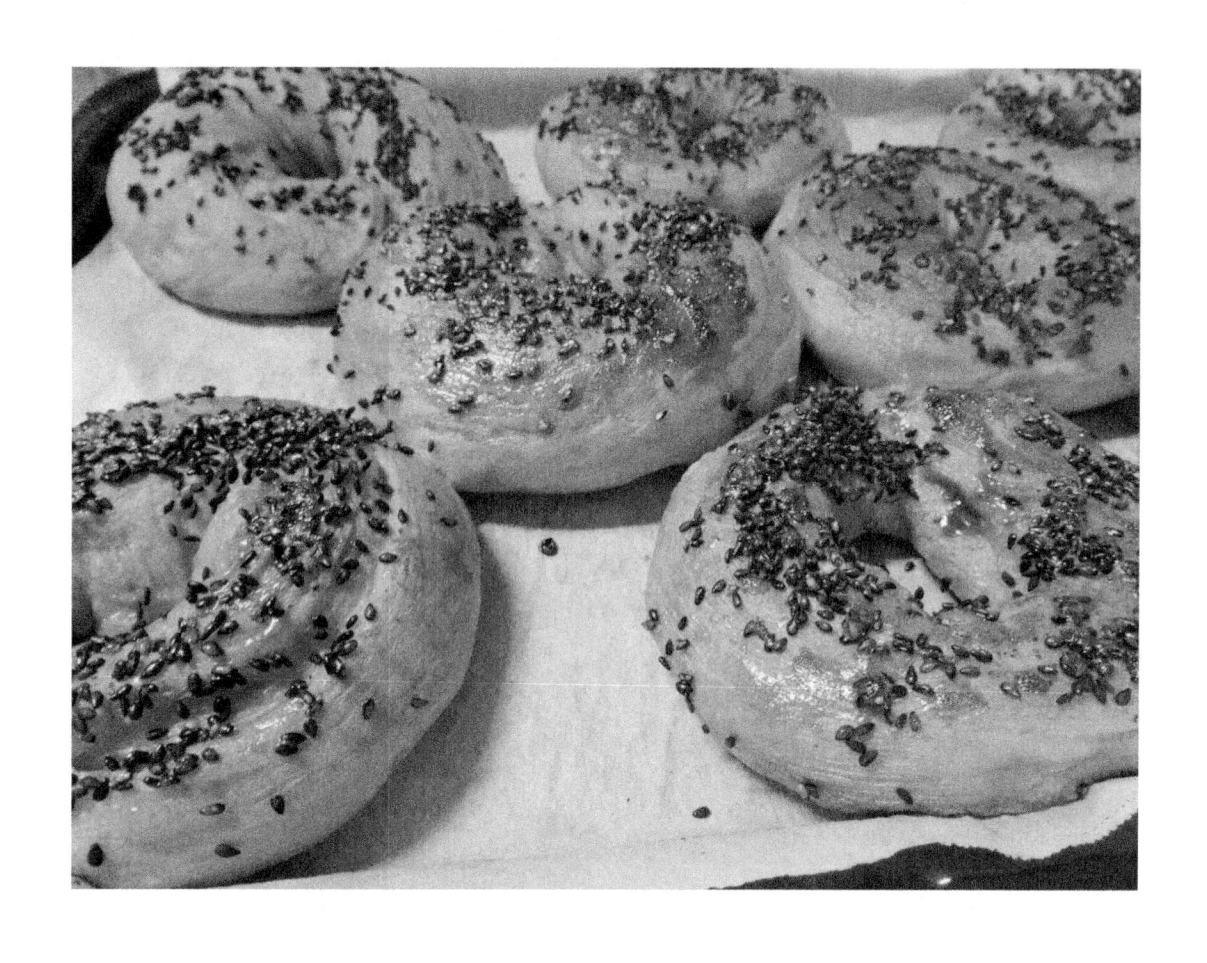

Pizza Bagels

Yields: 10 bagels

Nutrition Facts: Amount per serving (1 bagel)

- Carbohydrates – 5.7g
- Protein – 15.8g
- Total Fat – 12.6g
- Calories – 189

Ingredients:

a. 2 cups almond flour

b. 1 ½ cups whey isolate

c. 12 tbsp. water

d. 6 tbsp. tomato sauce, sugar-free

e. 4 tbsp. parmesan, grated

f. 1 tbsp. baking powder

g. ½ tbsp. xanthan gum

h. Parmesan and mozzarella, grated for topping

Directions:

1. Line a baking sheet with parchment paper and preheat your oven to 375° F (190° C).

2. Mix all the dry ingredients in a mixing bowl.

3. Add in the water and tomato sauce. Stir until you form a dough.

4. Divide the dough into 10 and shape them into bagels.

5. Place onto the baking sheet and top with grated cheese.

6. Bake the bagels for 20 minutes or until golden brown.

7. Let the bagels cool and serve.

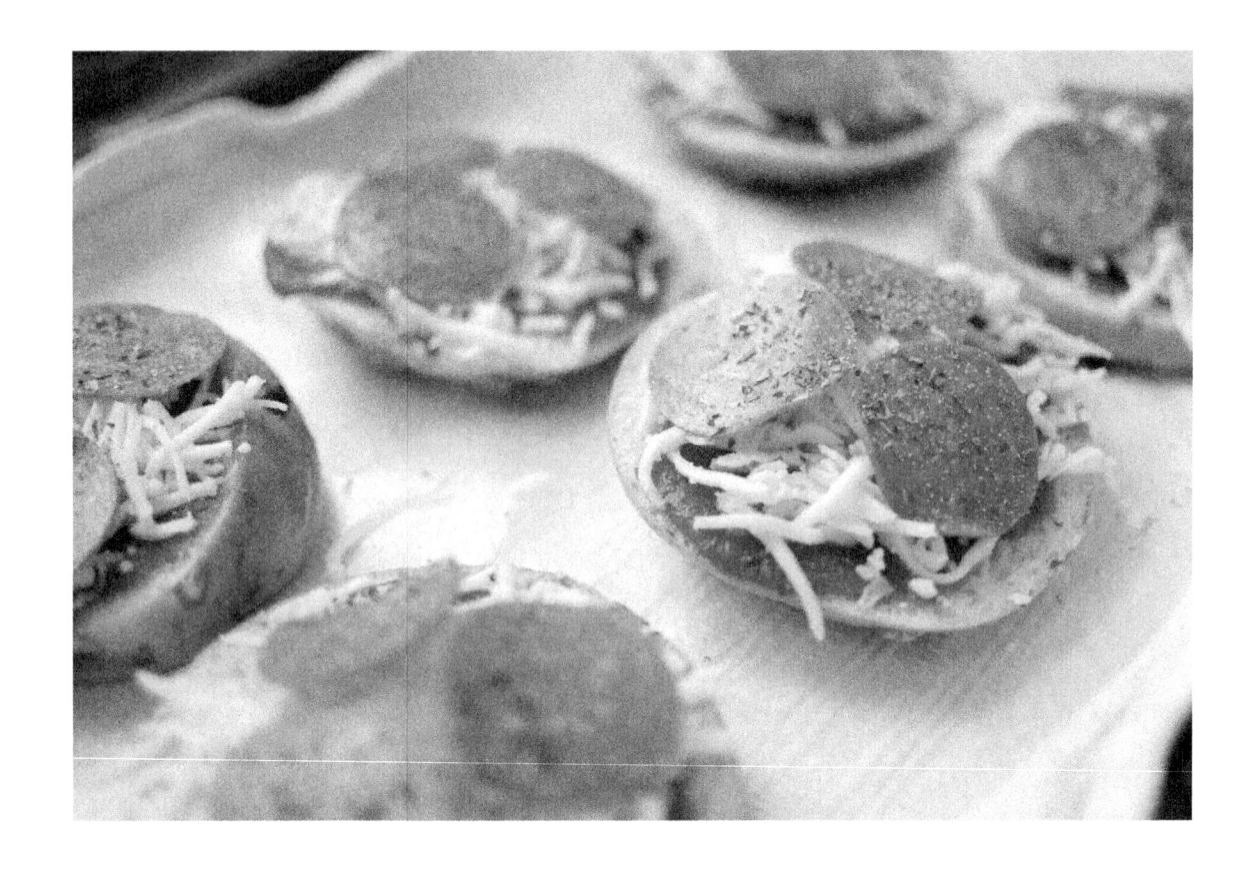

Rosemary Bagels

Yields: 4 bagels

Nutrition Facts: Amount per serving (1 bagel)

- Carbohydrates – 12g
- Protein – 13g
- Total Fat – 22.5g
- Calories – 285

Ingredients:

a. 1 ½ cups almond flour
b. ½ cup water, warm
c. 3 tbsp. psyllium husk powder
d. 1 tbsp. rosemary, chopped
e. ¾ tsp. xanthan gum
f. ¾ tsp. baking soda
g. ¼ tsp. salt
h. Avocado oil for greasing
i. 1 egg + 3 egg whites

Directions:

1. Preheat your oven to 250° F (120° C). Grease a 4-piece bagel mold (or a donut mold) with avocado oil.
2. In a mixing bowl, combine the xanthan gum, salt, baking soda, and almond flour.
3. Whisk the water and eggs in a separate bowl. Add in the psyllium husk and mix until smooth.
4. Combine the wet mixture to the dry mixture and mix well.
5. Press the mixture into the mold and top with chopped rosemary.
6. Bake for 45 minutes until
7. Remove the bagels form the mold, cool, and serve.

Cauliflower Bagels

Yields: 6 bagels

Nutrition Facts: Amount per serving (1 bagel)

- ➢ Carbohydrates – 11g
- ➢ Protein – 17g
- ➢ Total Fat – 13g
- ➢ Calories – 231

Ingredients:

a. 4 cups cauliflower, finely chopped

b. 2 cups mozzarella, shredded part-skim low moisture

c. ½ cup coconut flour

d. ½ cup almond flour, superfine

e. 2 tsp. baking powder

f. 3 large eggs

g. Everything bagel seasoning (store-bought or homemade) for topping

h. 1 egg, beaten for egg wash

Directions:

1. Use a cheesecloth to wring out all the moisture from the cauliflower. The cauliflower should be reduced to 1 ½ cup.
2. Preheat your oven to 400° F (200° C) and line a baking sheet with parchment paper.
3. Combine the dried cauliflower with the rest of the ingredients except the beaten egg and seasoning. Mix everything well.
4. Divide the batter into 6. Press one portion into ½ measuring cups tightly. Remove the batter portion from the cup onto the baking sheet. Press a hole in the center and stretch to make it bigger. Repeat for all batter portions to make the bagels.
5. Brush the egg wash on the bagels and sprinkle a generous amount of everything bagel seasoning.
6. Bake for 22 minutes or until the bagels turn dark golden brown. It's done when the bagels bounce back when pressed.
7. Let the bagels cool for a while before serving. They can also be refrigerated or frozen.

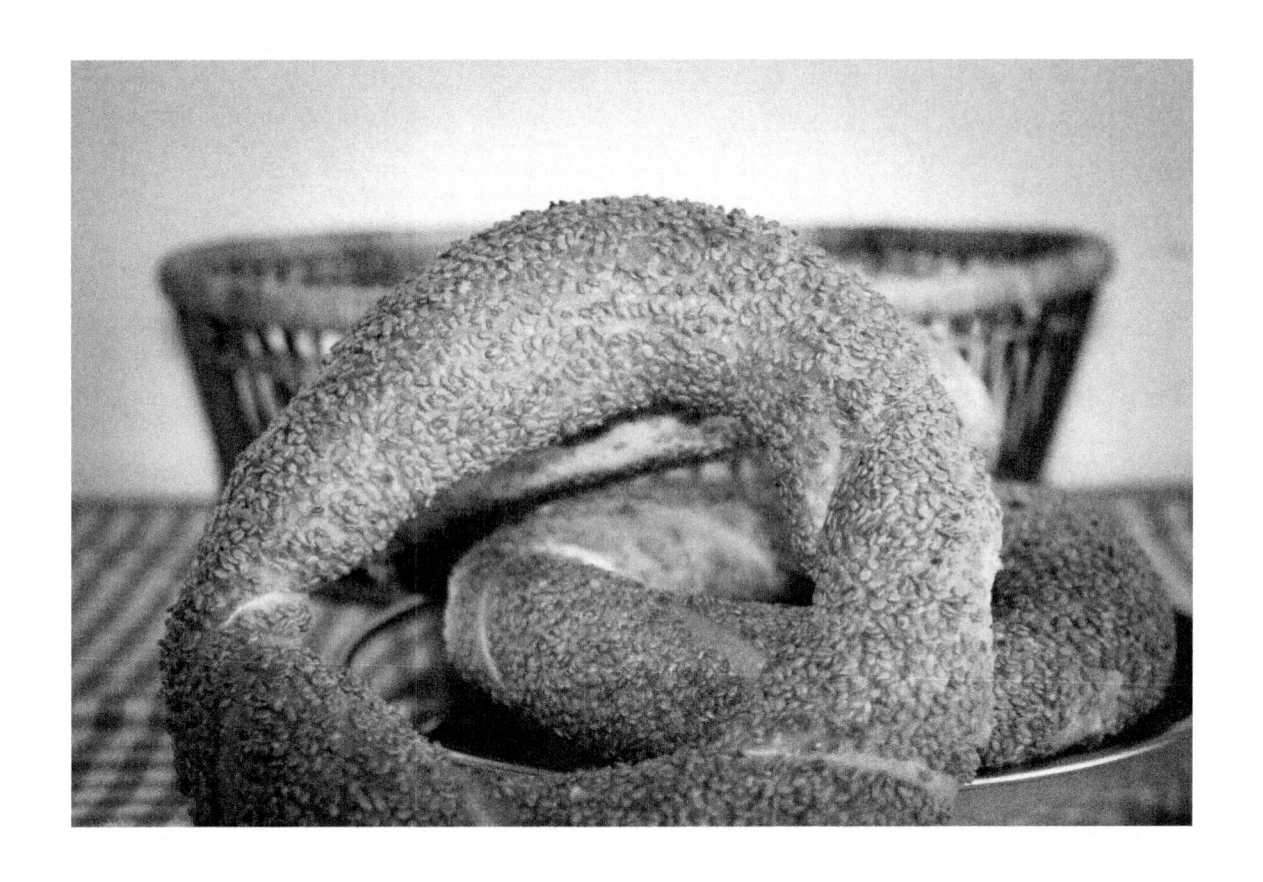

Jalapeno Bagels

Yields: 6 bagels

Nutrition Facts: Amount per serving (1 bagel)

- Carbohydrates – 6g
- Protein – 6g
- Total Fat – 22g
- Calories – 273

Ingredients:

a. 2 oz. cream cheese
b. 2 cups mozzarella, grated
c. 1 cup cheddar, grated
d. 1 cup almond flour
e. 1 tsp. baking powder
f. 3 jalapenos, deseeded and sliced thinly (set aside a few slices for topping)
g. 2 eggs

Directions:

1. Grease a bagel pan (or a donut pan) and preheat your oven to 400° F (200° C).

2. Mix the baking powder and almond flour in a bowl. Add the jalapenos and eggs and mix well.
3. Melt the cream cheese and mozzarella in the microwave for 1 minute. Give it a good stir and melt it for another minute.
4. Add the almond mixture to the cheese and stir well until you form a dough.
5. Divide the dough into 6 pieces and shape into bagels. Top them with jalapenos and cheddar.
6. Bake for 20 to 30 minutes or until golden brown.
7. Cool the bagels before serving.

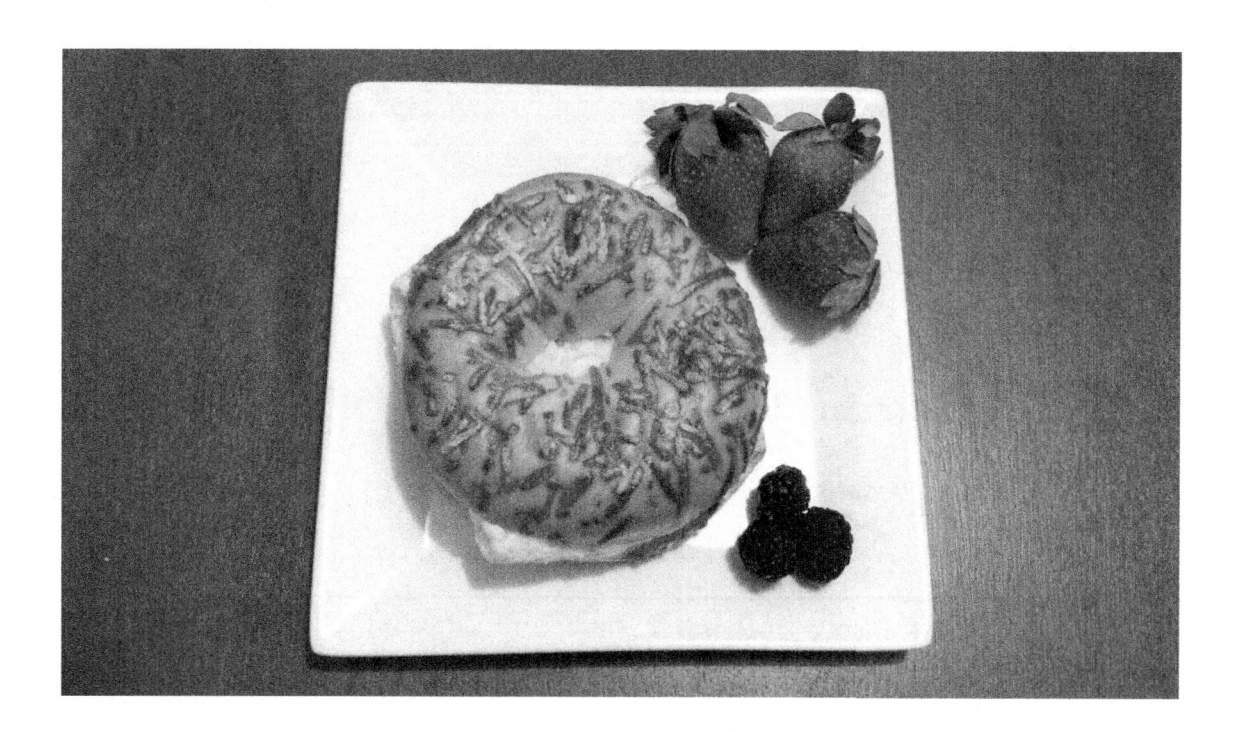

Blueberry Cheesecake Bagels

Yields: 12 bagels

Nutrition Facts: Amount per serving (1 bagel)

- ➢ Carbohydrates – 3.3g
- ➢ Protein – 3.8g
- ➢ Total Fat – 5.1g
- ➢ Calories – 68

Ingredients:

a. 2 oz. cream cheese
b. 2 ½ cups mozzarella, grated
c. ¾ cup nut flour
d. ¾ cup almond flour
e. ½ cup blueberries, fresh
f. 1 tbsp. baking powder
g. 2 tsp. Erythritol sweetener, divided
h. 2 eggs
i. 1 egg, beaten for egg wash

Directions:

1. Preheat the oven to 400° F (200° C). Prepare a baking sheet and line it with parchment paper.
2. Melt the cream cheese and mozzarella in the microwave until well-melted. Stir every after 30 seconds to avoid crusting the cheese. Once the cheese is melted, add in 2 eggs and mix well.
3. In a different bowl, combine the baking powder, almond flour, and 1 tsp. Erythritol. Then, set aside.
4. Combine the flour and cheese mixtures together until you form a dough.
5. Knead the dough until all the ingredients are well-incorporated.
6. Fold in the blueberries carefully.
7. Divide the dough into 8 and form into bagels. Place them on the baking sheet.
8. Brush the bagels with the egg wash. Sprinkle the tops with the remaining Erythritol.
9. Bake for about 10 to 14 minutes or until the bagels become light brown.
10. Remove from the oven and cool before serving.

Cinnamon Bagels

Yields: 6 bagels

Nutrition Facts: Amount per serving (1 bagel)

- Carbohydrates – 17.8g
- Protein – 25.4g
- Total Fat – 19.9g
- Calories – 317

Ingredients:

a. 2 oz. cream cheese

b. 2 ½ cups mozzarella, grated

c. 1 ¾ cups almond flour

d. ¼ cup coconut flour

e. 3 tbsp. Monkfruit, divided

f. 1 tbsp. cinnamon, divided

g. 2 tsp. cream of tartar

h. 1 tsp. baking

i. 2 large eggs

j. 1 egg, beaten for egg wash

Directions:

1. Place parchment paper on a baking sheet and preheat the oven to 400° F (200° C).
2. Combine the almond and coconut flours, cream of tartar, baking soda, 1 tsp. cinnamon, and 1 tbsp. Monkfruit in a large mixing bowl
3. Melt the mozzarella and cream cheese in the microwave for 1 minute. Take out the cheese and stir. Melt again for 30 seconds more and stir after.
4. In a separate bowl, whisk 2 eggs and add it to the flour mixture. Add in the cheese as well and knead very well until you form a dough.
5. Divide the dough into 6 and form them into bagels. Brush on the egg wash and sprinkle the remaining Monkfruit and cinnamon on top of the bagels.
6. Place them on the baking sheet and bake for about 12 to 14 minutes. Monitor the bagels to make sure that the cinnamon doesn't burn.
7. Take out the bagels and transfer to a cooling rack. Cool the bagels for about 15 minutes to let the remaining heat continue cooking the inside before serving.

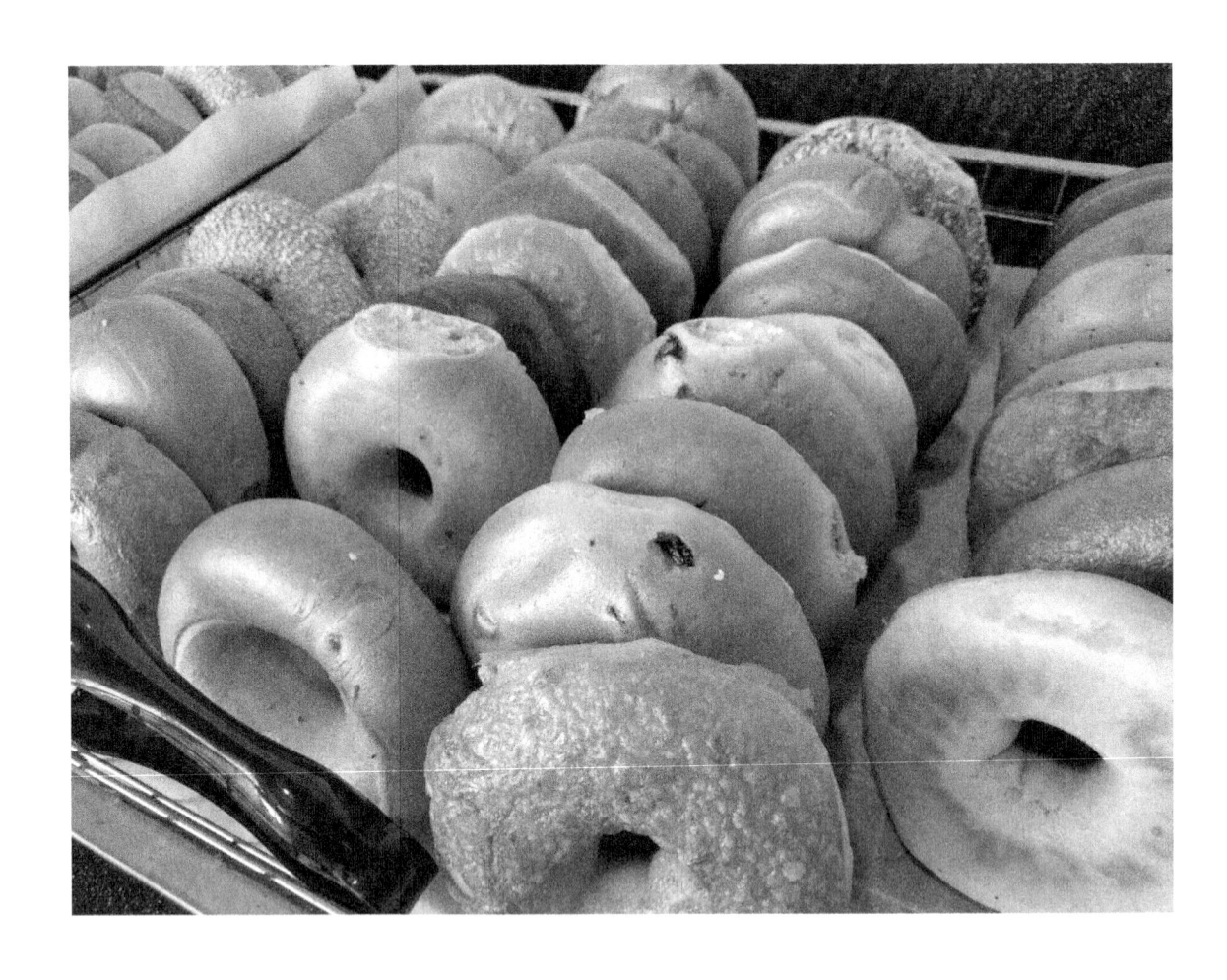

CHAPTER 4

Keto Pizza

Fathead Pizza Crust

Yields: 1 pizza (8 slices)

Nutrition Facts: Amount per serving (1 slice of the crust)

- ➤ Carbohydrates – 5g
- ➤ Protein – 14g
- ➤ Total Fat – 19g
- ➤ Calories – 249

Ingredients: (Crust)

a. 2 cups mozzarella, grated
b. 1 cup almond flour
c. 2 tbsp. cream cheese
d. 1 tsp. baking powder
e. 1 tsp. Italian seasoning
f. 1 tsp. garlic powder
g. 1 egg

(Toppings: based on your preference)

    a. Cheese: mozzarella, feta, parmesan, etc.

    b. Meats: beef, chicken, turkey, etc.

    c. Vegetables: peppers, onions, olives, etc.

    d. Sauce: tomato sauce (sugar-free), ranch, olive oil, etc.

Directions:

1. Preheat the oven to 450° F (230° C).
2. Melt the cream cheese and mozzarella in the microwave for 45 seconds.
3. Add the remaining crust ingredients together to the cheese and combine well.
4. Place the dough in between two sheets of parchment paper.
5. Flatten the dough with a rolling pin until it's ¼-inch thick. Then, shape it with your hands if desired.
6. Transfer the pizza to a baking sheet. Bake for 10 minutes.
7. Without turning the oven off, take out the pizza and put on your chosen toppings.
8. Put the pizza back in the oven and bake for 5 minutes more or until the cheese topping melts.
9. Slice into 8 pieces and serve.

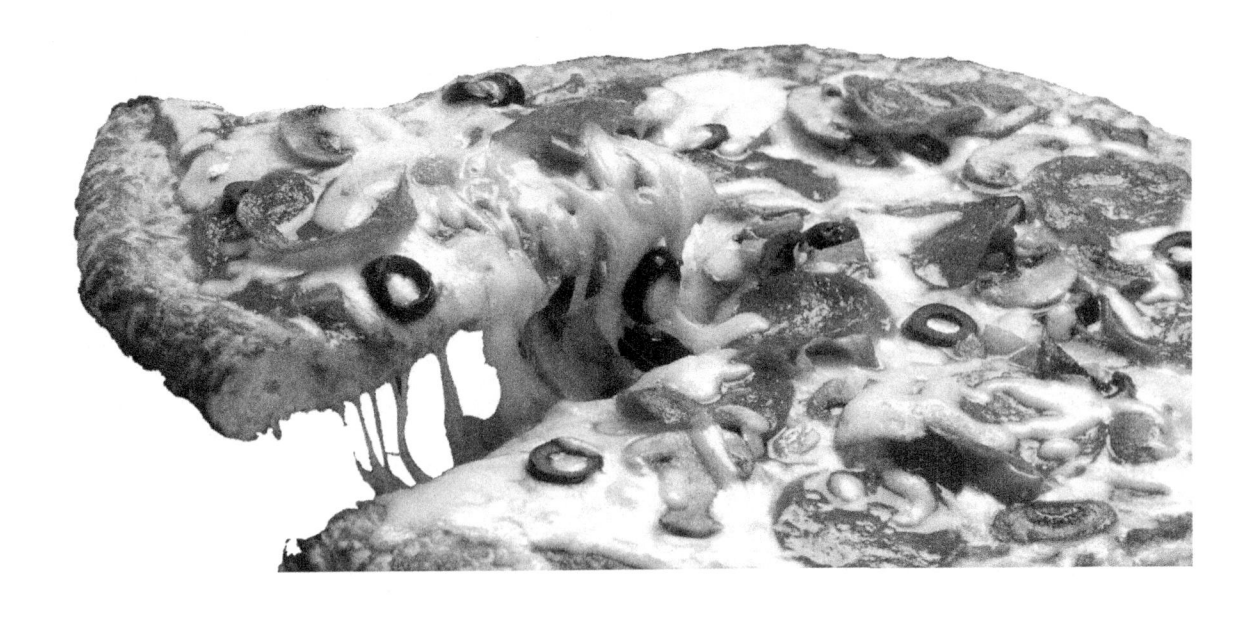

Easy Mozzarella Crust Pizza

Yields: 2 pizzas (8 slices)

Nutrition Facts: Amount per serving (1 slice)

- Carbohydrates – 1.5g
- Protein – 13.25g
- Total Fat – 22.5g
- Calories – 260

Ingredients: (Crust)

a. 6 oz. mozzarella, grated
b. 4 eggs

(Topping)

a. 5 oz. any cheese you prefer, grated
b. 1 ½ oz. pepperoni
c. 3 tbsp. tomato sauce, sugar-free
d. 1 tsp. oregano, dried
e. Olives, sliced

Directions:

1. Preheat the oven to 400° F (200° C). Line a baking sheet with parchment paper.

2. Combine the eggs and cheese in a mixing bowl.

3. Spread the egg and cheese mixture on the baking sheet. Divide the mixture into two and make 2 round circles.

4. Bake for 15 minutes or until the crusts turn golden brown. Take them out and cool for about a minute.

5. Increase the oven's temperature to 225° C or 450° F.

6. Evenly spread the tomato sauce over the crusts. Then, top with oregano, cheese, pepperoni, and olives.

7. Put the pizza back into the oven and bake for about 5 to 10 minutes. Let the pizzas cool. Slice each pizza into 4 pieces.

White Pizza

Yields: 1 pizza (8 slices)

Nutrition Facts: Amount per serving (1 slice)

- ➤ Carbohydrates – 2.75g
- ➤ Protein – 9g
- ➤ Total Fat – 25g
- ➤ Calories – 273

Ingredients: (Crust)

a. ¾ cup almond flour

b. ½ cup mayonnaise

c. 1 tbsp. psyllium husk powder, ground

d. 1 tsp. baking powder

e. ½ tsp. salt

f. 2 eggs

(Topping)

a. 2 oz. parmesan

b. ¾ cup any cheese you prefer, grated

c. ½ cup sour cream

d. 1 tsp. rosemary, fresh or dried

e. ½ tsp. black pepper, ground

f. 2 eggs

Directions:

1. Line a large baking sheet with parchment paper and preheat your oven to 350° F (175° C).

2. Combine the mayonnaise and eggs in a mixing bowl. Then, add in the rest of the crust ingredients and let it sit for about 5 minutes.

3. Spread out the pizza batter on the baking sheet. Your rolling pin should be oiled so the batter won't stick to it. Shape it into a round circle that should only be ½-inch thick.

4. Bake the crust for 10 minutes or until light golden brown.

5. Don't turn off the oven and take the crust out of the oven and flip it over.

6. Spread the sour cream on the crust. Top with grated cheese you prefer. Then, rosemary and pepper.

7. Bake the pizza for another 5 to 10 minutes. Monitor is constantly and don't let the edges brown too much.

8. Take it out of the oven and sprinkle parmesan over the pizza. Slice into 8 pieces and serve.

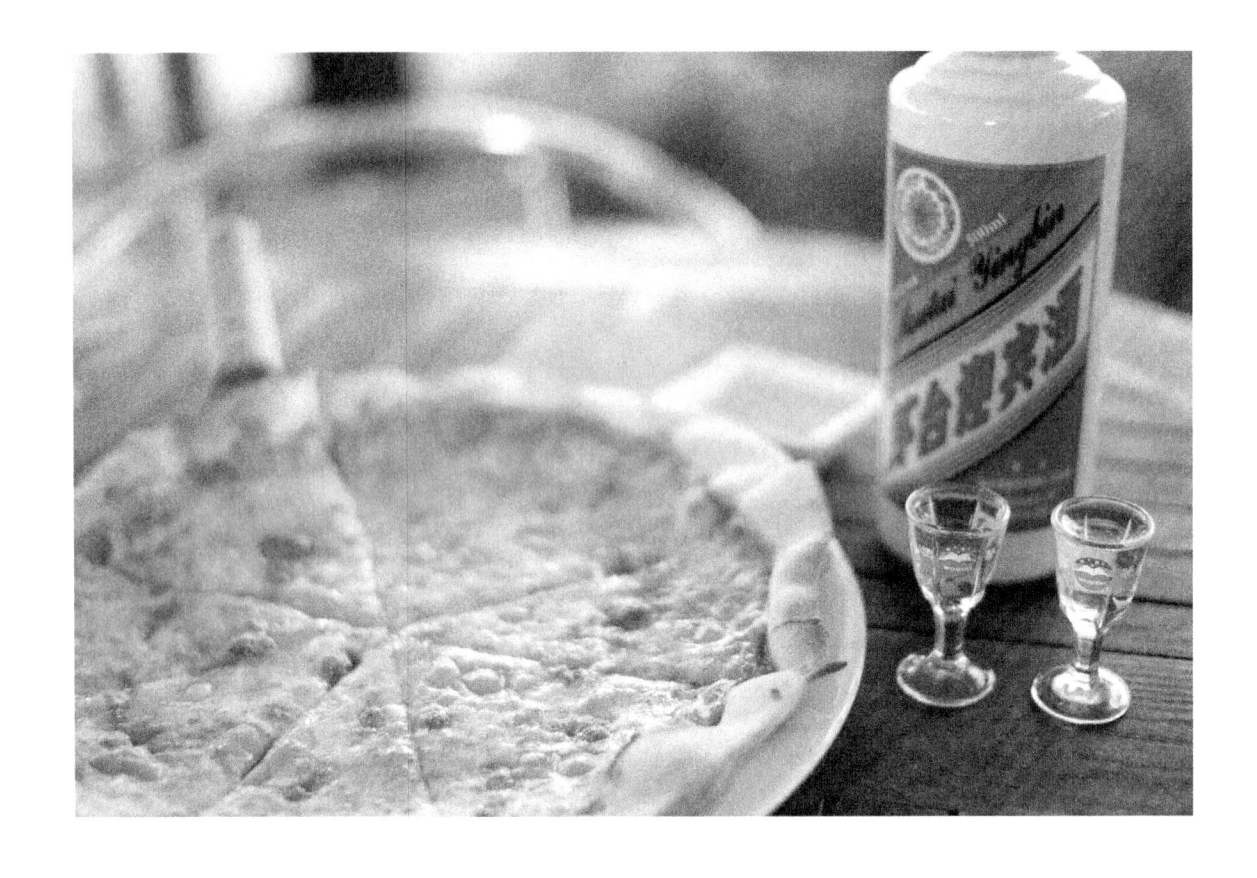

Thin Crust Pizza

Yields: 1 pizza (8 slices)

Nutrition Facts: Amount per serving (1 slice)

- ➢ Carbohydrates – 4g
- ➢ Protein – 1g
- ➢ Total Fat – 4g
- ➢ Calories – 54

Ingredients: (Crust)

a. 1 cup almond flour

b. ¼ cup coconut flour

c. 1 ½ tbsp. vinegar

d. 1 tbsp. olive oil

e. 2 tsp. Italian seasoning

f. 1 ½ tsp. xanthan gum

g. 1 tsp. garlic powder

h. 1 tsp. salt

i. 1 tsp. yeast

j. 1 egg, beaten + 1 tbsp. water

(Topping)

a. ¼ cup pesto

b. ½ cup mozzarella, fresh

c. 2 sun-dried tomatoes

Directions:

1. Preheat the oven to 425° F (220° C).
2. Combine the ingredients except for the egg mixture and olive oil in a bowl.
3. Add the egg mixture to the mixture in small batches stirring in between. Continue mixing until you form a dough.
4. Place the dough in between two sheets or parchment paper and flatten with a rolling pin. Roll it out into a 12-inch circle.
5. Remove the top parchment paper and transfer the dough onto a baking sheet.
6. Brush the dough with olive oil. Bake for 5-7 minutes.
7. Take the crust out and lower the oven's temperature to 350° F (175° C).
8. Place the toppings on the pizza and place it back in the oven. Bake until the cheese melts.
9. Slice into 8 pieces and serve.

Chicken Barbecue Pizza

Yields: 1 pizza (4 slices)

Nutrition Facts: Amount per serving (1 slice)

- Carbohydrates – 9.2g
- Protein – 24.5 g
- Total Fat – 24.5g
- Calories – 357

Ingredients: (Crust)

a. 6 tbsp. parmesan
b. 3 tbsp. psyllium husk powder
c. 1 ½ tsp. Italian seasoning
d. 6 large eggs
e. Salt and pepper to taste

(Topping)

a. 6 oz. rotisserie chicken, shredded
b. 4 oz. cheddar
c. 4 tbsp. barbecue sauce, low-carb
d. 4 tbsp. tomato sauce, sugar-free
e. 1 tbsp. mayonnaise

Directions:

1. Preheat the oven to 425° F (220° C). Combine all the crust ingredients until thick.
2. Spread the crust batter onto a large lined baking sheet. Shape it into a round circle. Place on the oven's top rack and bake for 10 minutes.
3. Flip the pizza crust and evenly place the toppings.
4. Broil for 3 minutes or until the cheddar melts. Slice into 4 pieces and serve.

Portobello Mushroom Personal Pizzas

Yields: 4 personal pizzas

Nutrition Facts: Amount per serving (1 personal pizza)

- Carbohydrates – 5.23g
- Protein – 10.3g
- Total Fat – 31.58g
- Calories – 338.75

Ingredients:

a. 4 oz. fresh mozzarella, cubed
b. 4 large Portobello caps
c. 1 medium tomato, thinly sliced to about 12 slices
d. ¼ cup basil, chopped
e. 6 tbsp. olive oil
f. 20 slices pepperoni
g. Salt and pepper to taste

Directions:

1. Scrape the mushrooms' innards and meat out until you're left with only the shells.
2. Use 3 tbsp. olive oil to rub the tops of the mushroom shells. Season with salt and pepper. Broil for 4-5 minutes.

3. Flip the shells over and repeat step 2 on the other side of the shells.

4. Top the mushrooms with the rest of the ingredients.

5. Broil again until the cheese melts. Let cool then serve.

Bell Pepper & Basil Pizza

Yields: 2 pizzas (8 slices)

Nutrition Facts: Amount per serving (1 slice)

- Carbohydrates – 6.25g
- Protein – 11.13g
- Total Fat – 15.66g
- Calories – 205.75

Ingredients: (Crust)

a. 6 oz. mozzarella, melted
b. ½ cup almond flour
c. 2 tbsp. cream cheese
d. 2 tbsp. fresh parmesan
e. 2 tbsp. psyllium husk powder
f. 1 tbsp. Italian seasoning
g. ½ tsp. pepper
h. ½ tsp. salt
i. 1 large egg

(Topping)

a. 4 oz. cheddar, grated
b. ¼ cup tomato sauce, sugar-free

c. 1 medium tomato, sliced

   d. 2/3 bell pepper, chopped

   e. 3 tbsp. fresh basil, chopped

Directions:

1. Preheat the oven to 400° F (200° C).
2. Combine all the crust ingredients and mix well.
3. Divide the dough into 2. Roll out the dough and form round circles.
4. Bake for about 10 minutes.
5. Remove from the oven and place the toppings. Bake for 8 minutes more or until the cheddar melts.
6. Cut each pizza into 4. Serve.

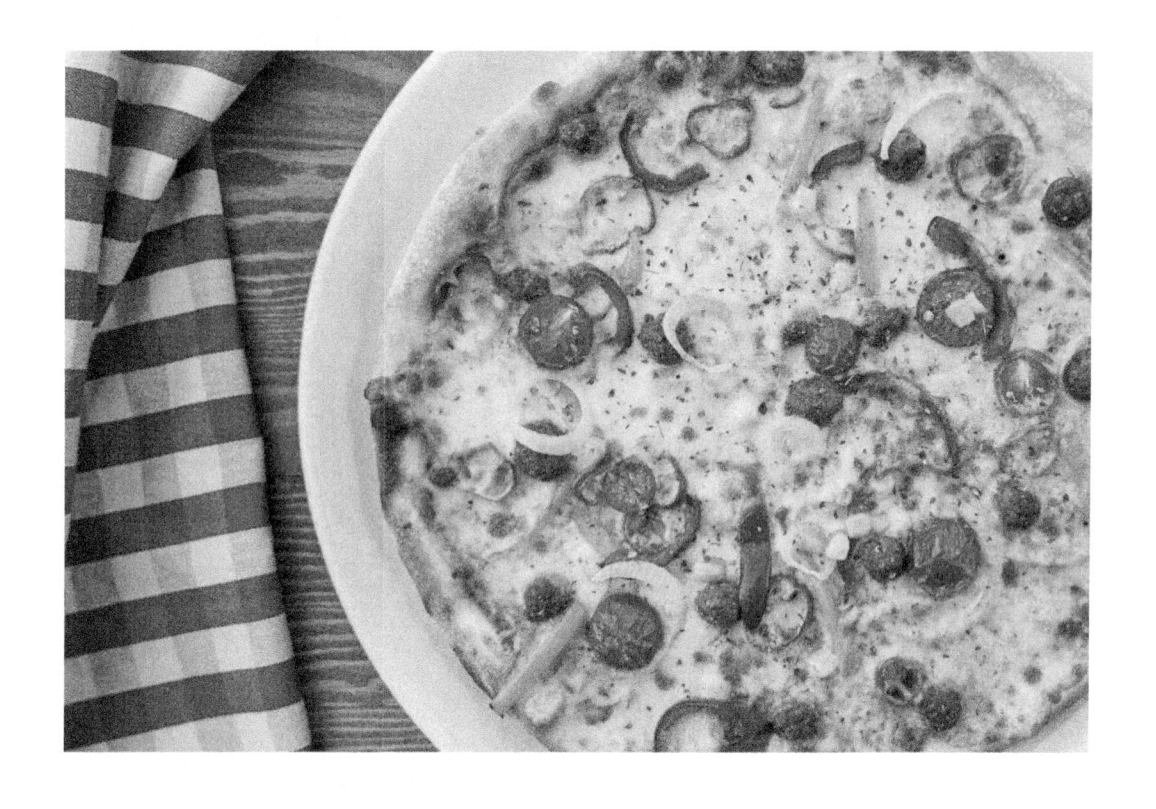

Buffalo Chicken Pizza

Yields: 1 pizza (8 slices)

Nutrition Facts: Amount per serving (1 slice)

- Carbohydrates – 1.05g
- Protein – 13.83g
- Total Fat – 12.88g
- Calories – 172

Ingredients:

a. 1 lb. chicken thighs, boneless and skinless, ground
b. 1 oz. blue cheese, crumbled
c. 1 cup whole-milk mozzarella, grated
d. 3 tbsp. cayenne pepper sauce
e. 2 tbsp. butter
f. 1 tbsp. sour cream
g. 1 tsp. oregano, dried
h. ¼ tsp. black pepper
i. ¼ tsp. salt
j. 1 celery stalk (64g), finely diced
k. 1 green onion stalk (12g), chopped
l. 1 large egg

Directions:

1. Preheat the oven to 400° F (200° C). Line a 14-inch pizza pan with parchment paper.
2. Combine the chicken, ½ cup of the mozzarella, oregano, egg, salt, and pepper and mix well.
3. Spread the chicken batter onto the pizza pan. It should be ¼-inch thick.
4. Bake for about 25 minutes until the top has started to brown.
5. In a skillet, melt the butter and cook the celery until brown.
6. Combine the pepper sauce and sour cream in a bowl. Set aside.
7. Take out the crust. Spread the sauce over the crust. Layer the celery, blue cheese, and remaining mozzarella on the crust.
8. Bake for 10 minutes more or until the cheese melts and browns. Broil the last few minutes.
9. Drizzle pepper sauce and sprinkle green onions before slicing.

Pan-Fried Pizza Margherita

Yields: 1 pizza

Nutrition Facts: Amount per serving (1 pizza)

- ➢ Carbohydrates – 3.5g
- ➢ Protein – 27g
- ➢ Total Fat – 35g
- ➢ Calories – 459

Ingredients: (Crust)

a. 2 tbsp. parmesan
b. 1 tbsp. psyllium husk powder
c. ½ tsp. Italian seasoning
d. A dash of salt
e. 2 tsp. oil for frying
f. 2 eggs

(Topping)

a. 1.5 oz. mozzarella
b. 3 tbsp. tomato sauce, sugar-free
c. 1 tbsp. fresh basil, chopped

Directions:

1. Combine all the crust ingredients in a bowl. You can use an immersion blender to make sure everything's mixed well.
2. Heat the oil in a pan. Spoon the batter in the pad and spread out to form a round crust.
3. Cook until the edges turn brown. Then, flip the crust and cook for an additional 30-60 seconds.
4. Remove from the heat then place the toppings.
5. Broil the pizza or until the cheese starts to melt and bubble. Slice before serving.

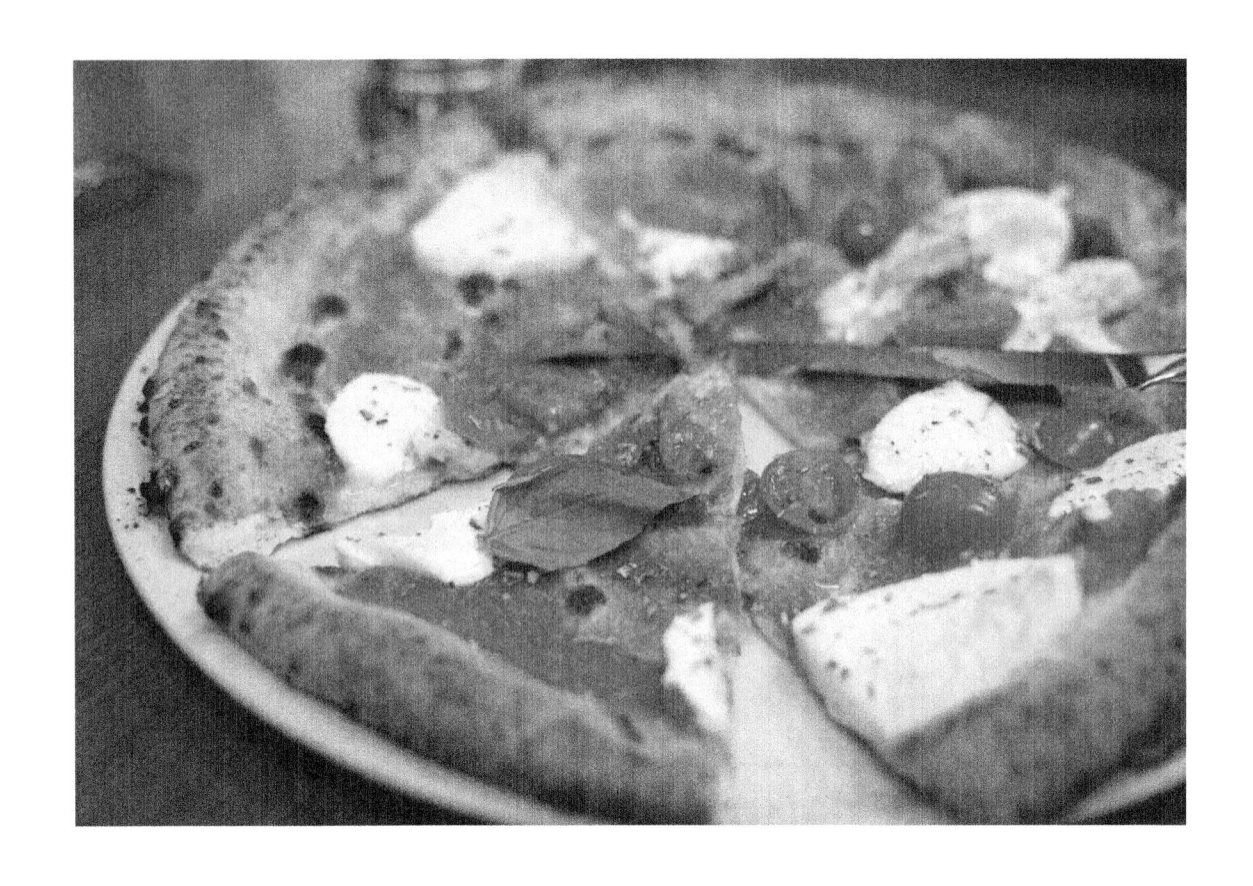

Cinnamon Pizza

Yields: 1 pizza (8 slices)

Nutrition Facts: Amount per serving (1 slice)

- ➢ Carbohydrates – 2g
- ➢ Protein – 2g
- ➢ Total Fat – 9g
- ➢ Calories – 93

Ingredients: (Crust)

a. ¾ cup almond flour
b. 2 tbsp. flax meal
c. 1 tbsp. ghee
d. 1 tbsp. cinnamon powder
e. 1 tsp. baking powder
f. A dash of Erythritol
g. 1 egg, beaten

(Topping)

a. 2 tbsp. coconut cream
b. 1 tbsp. ghee, melted
c. 1 tsp. cinnamon powder
d. Erythritol to taste

Directions:

1. Preheat the oven to 400° F (200° C).
2. Mix all the crust ingredients and form a dough. Roll and flatten it out into a round circle.
3. Bake for about 15 minutes. Flip the crust and bake for 5 minutes more.
4. Combine the cinnamon and ghee and mix well. Spread it on the crust.
5. Freeze the pizza for 1 hour.
6. Combine the Erythritol and coconut cream and place in the fridge for 30 minutes.
7. Spread the coconut cream onto the pizza. Slice into 8 pieces and serve.

Fruit Dessert Pizza

Yields: 1 pizza (8 slices)

Nutrition Facts: Amount per serving (1 slice)

- ➤ Carbohydrates – 6.9g
- ➤ Protein – 5.4g
- ➤ Total Fat – 26.9g
- ➤ Calories – 286

Ingredients: (Crust)

- g. 2 oz. cream cheese, softened
- h. 1/3 cup Erythritol sweetener
- i. 2 tbsp. butter, unsalted, softened
- j. 1 tsp. vanilla extract
- k. 8 eggs

(Topping)

- d. 2 oz. cream cheese, softened
- e. ½ cup heavy whipping cream
- f. 1/4 cup Erythritol sweetener
- g. 2 tbsp. butter, unsalted, softened

h. 1 tsp. vanilla extract

i. 1 cup strawberries, quartered

j. 3/4 cup blueberries

Directions:

6. Line a 112-inch pizza pan with parchment paper and grease with non-stick spray. Preheat your oven to 350° F (180° C).
7. Combine the butter, vanilla, cream cheese, and eythritol in a bowl and mix well. Then, mix in the egg. Finally, add the almond flour until smooth.
8. Pour and even out the batter onto the pizza pan.
9. Bake for 20-24 minutes until it turns golden brown.
10. Take out the pizza and set aside to cool.
11. Combine all the topping ingredients except for the whipping cream and berries. Once mixed, add the whipping cream. The volume should be doubled.
12. Spread the frosting over the crust evenly. Top with the fruits and slice into 8 pieces.

CHAPTER 5

Keto Muffins

Quick-and-Easy Muffins

Yields: 1 muffin

Nutrition Facts: Amount per serving (1 muffin)

- Carbohydrates – 5g
- Protein – 7g
- Total Fat – 6g
- Calories – 113

Ingredients:

a. 2 tsp. coconut flour (amount may depend on brand)
b. A pinch of salt
c. A pinch of baking soda
d. 1 egg

Directions:

1. Grease a coffee mug or ramekin dish with butter or coconut oil.

2. Mix all the ingredients in the mug or dish until it's free of lumps.

3. Set the microwave on high and cook the muffin for 45 minutes. (If using an oven, cook for 12 minutes at 400° F (200° C).)

4. Remove from the dish and serve.

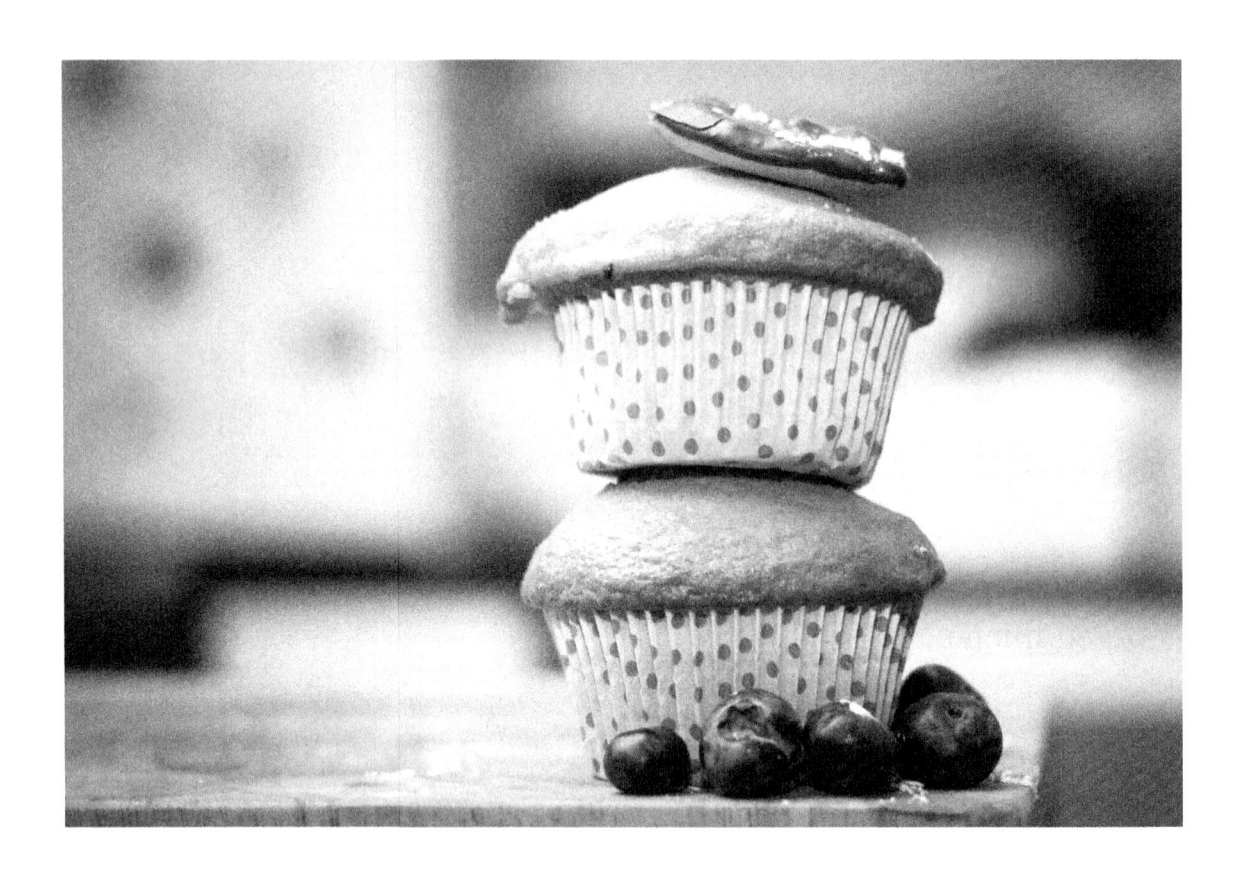

Quick-and-Easy Cinnamon Muffins

Yields: 1 muffin

Nutrition Facts: Amount per serving (1 muffin)

- Carbohydrates – 11.1g
- Protein – 7.01g
- Total Fat – 6.03g
- Calories – 119

Ingredients:

a. All the ingredients for the **Quick-and-Easy Muffins**
b. 1 tsp. Stevia
c. 1 tsp. cinnamon
d. Butter, Stevia, and cinnamon for topping

Directions:

1. Follow the directions for the **Quick-and-Easy Muffins** recipe. But, add the Stevia and cinnamon in the batter.
2. Before serving, brush the top with butter and sprinkle Stevia and cinnamon.

Quick-and-Easy Feta & Cheese Muffins

Yields: 1 muffin

Nutrition Facts: Amount per serving (1 muffin)

- Carbohydrates – 5.18g
- Protein – 7.45g
- Total Fat – 6.6g
- Calories – 121

Ingredients:

a. All the ingredients for the **Quick-and-Easy Muffins**
b. 2 tbsp. feta, grated
c. 1 tbsp. spinach

Directions:

1. Follow the directions for the **Quick-and-Easy Muffins** recipe. But, add the spinach and feta in the batter.

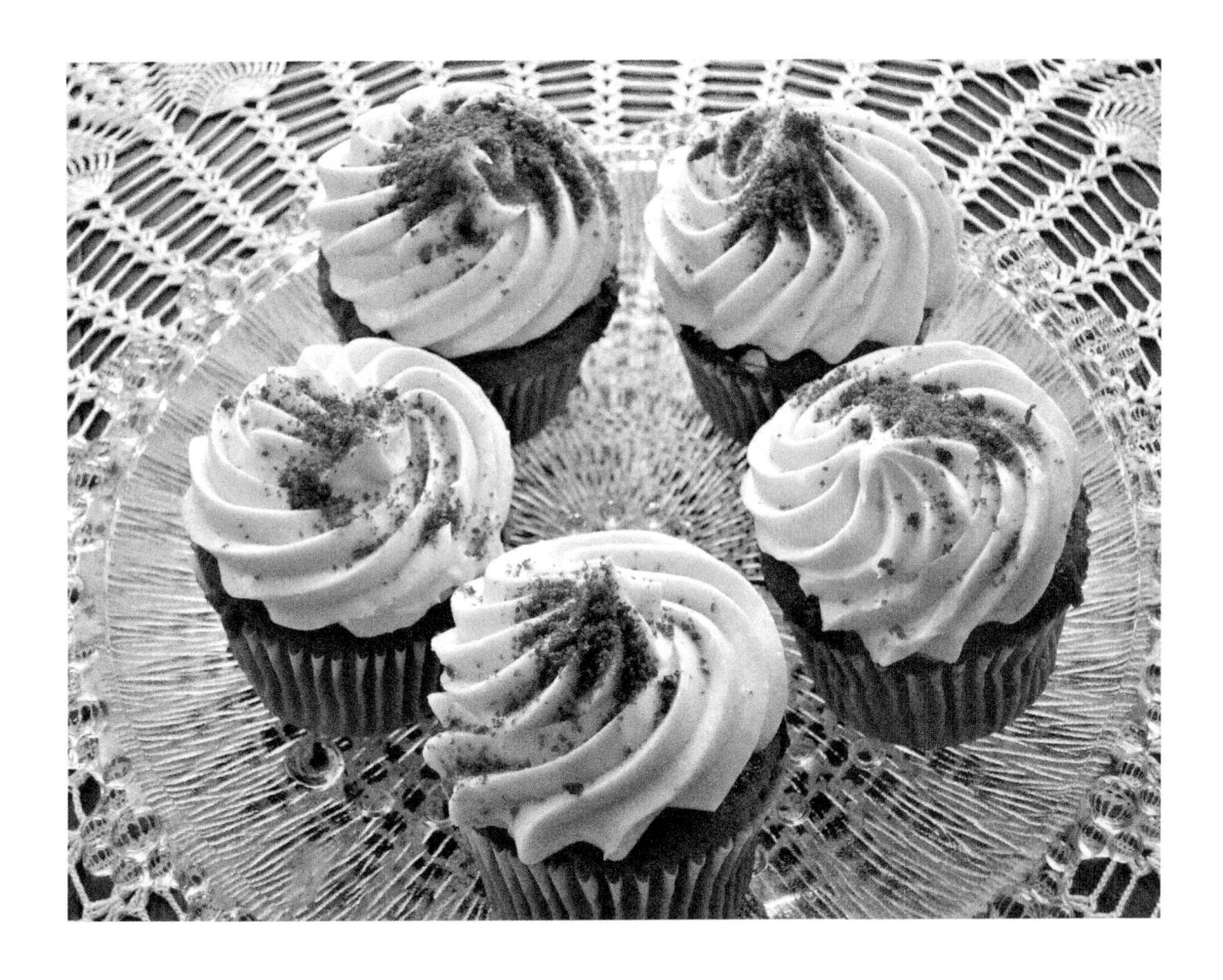

Quick-and-Easy Feta & Cheese Muffins

Yields: 1 muffin

Nutrition Facts: Amount per serving (1 muffin)

- Carbohydrates – 5.18g
- Protein – 7.45g
- Total Fat – 6.6g
- Calories – 121

Ingredients:

d. All the ingredients for the **Quick-and-Easy Muffins**
e. 2 tbsp. feta, grated
f. 1 tbsp. spinach

Directions:

1. Follow the directions for the **Quick-and-Easy Muffins** recipe. But, add the spinach and feta in the batter.

Cheesy Herbed Muffins

Yields: 8 muffins

Nutrition Facts: Amount per serving (1 muffin)

- Carbohydrates – 5g
- Protein – 7g
- Total Fat – 20g
- Calories – 216

Ingredients:

a. 1 cup blanched almond flour, superfine
b. ½ cup sharp cheddar, grated
c. 1/3 cup unsweetened almond milk
d. 6 tbsp. butter, melted
e. 3 tbsp. coconut flour
f. 2 tsp. baking powder
g. 1 tsp. Erythritol sweetener
h. ¾ tsp. kosher salt
i. ½ tsp. fresh thyme
j. ¼ tsp. garlic powder
k. ¼ tsp. xanthan gum
l. 2 eggs

Directions:

1. Preheat your oven to 375° F (190° C). Grease an 8-piece muffin tin.
2. Combine all the ingredients together. Mix until well-combined.
3. Scoop the batter into the muffin tin evenly.
4. Bake for about 22 minutes or do the toothpick test to know when it's done.
5. Let the muffins cool before serving.

Egg Muffins

Yields: 12 muffins

Nutrition Facts: Amount per serving (2 muffins)

- Carbohydrates – 2g
- Protein – 23g
- Total Fat – 26g
- Calories – 336

Ingredients:

a. 6 oz. cheese, shredded

b. 5 oz. air-dried chorizo, chopped

c. 2 tbsp. pesto sauce

d. 2 scallion stalks, finely chopped

e. Salt and pepper to taste

f. 12 eggs

Directions:

1. Preheat your oven to 350° F (180° C). Use butter to grease your muffin tin.
2. Place the chorizo and scallions to the muffin tin's bottoms.
3. Whisk the eggs, salt, pepper, and pesto. Then, mix in the cheese.

4. Pour the batter in your muffin tip. Bake for about 15 minutes or more. To know if it's ready, do the toothpick test.
5. Let them cool for a bit before serving.

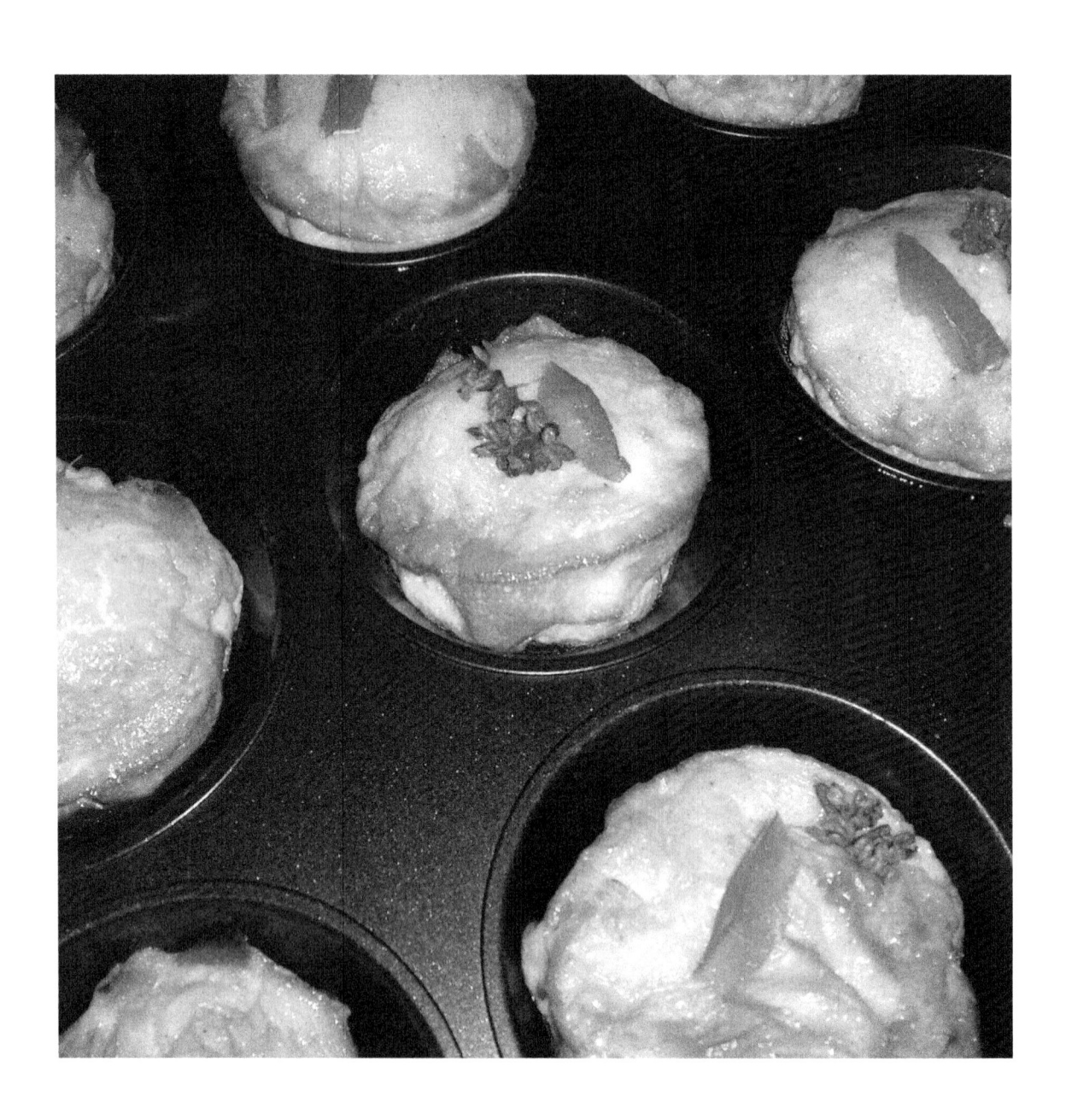

Ham & Zucchini Muffins

Yields: 12 muffins

Nutrition Facts: Amount per serving (1 muffin)

- ➢ Carbohydrates – 3g
- ➢ Protein – 9g
- ➢ Total Fat – 9g
- ➢ Calories – 135

Ingredients:

a. 1 cup almond flour

b. ½ cup parmesan

c. ¾ cup ham, diced

d. 1/3 cup sour cream

e. 1 zucchini, grated

f. 1 tsp. baking powder

g. ½ tsp. salt and pepper

h. 4 eggs

Directions:

1. Line a 12-piece muffin tin with muffin liners or small parchment paper sheets. Preheat the oven to 350° F (180° C).
2. Combine the cheese, eggs, ham, sour cream, and zucchini and mix well.
3. In a different bowl, mix the baking powder, flour, salt, and pepper.
4. Combine the wet and dry ingredients.
5. Scoop the batter into the muffin tin.
6. Bake for 35-40 minutes or until the tops become golden brown.
7. Cool for 5 minutes before serving.

Chicken Thyme Muffins

Yields: 12 muffins

Nutrition Facts: Amount per serving (1 muffin)

- Carbohydrates – 1g
- Protein – 9g
- Total Fat – 10g
- Calories – 125

Ingredients: (Muffin)

a. ½ cup coconut milk

b. 2 tbsp. thyme, chopped

c. 1 tbsp. coconut oil

d. 1 chicken breast, diced

e. 2 bacon slices, diced

f. 1 carrot, grated, wring out extra moisture

g. Salt and pepper to taste

h. 8 eggs

Directions:

1. Preheat your oven to 350° F (180° C).

2. Heat the coconut oil in a frying pan and cook the chicken and bacon until browned.

3. Transfer the chicken and bacon to a bowl. Add in the carrots and thyme. Season with salt and pepper. Mix everything well.
4. In another bowl, whisk the coconut cream and eggs. Then, pour into the chicken mixture.
5. Evenly spoon the mixture into a 12-piece muffin tin.
6. Bake for 25-30 minutes.
7. Let the muffins cool before serving.

Lemon Muffins

Yields: 6 muffins

Nutrition Facts: Amount per serving (1 muffin)

- Carbohydrates – 8g
- Protein – 8g
- Total Fat – 18g
- Calories – 219

Ingredients:

a. 1 ½ cups almond flour

b. ¼ cup heavy cream

c. 3 tbsp. Swerve or Xylitol sweetener

d. 1 lemon, juiced and zested

e. 1 tsp. baking powder

f. 2 eggs, yolks and whites separated

Directions:

1. Preheat the oven to 350° F (180° C) and line a muffin tin with parchment paper or muffin liners.
2. Combine the sweetener, lemon zest, yolks, and baking powder and mix well. Then, mix in the lemon juice and almond flour.
3. Whip the egg whites until you form soft peaks.

4. First, stir in a spoonful of egg whites to the flour mixture and stir. Then, carefully fold in the rest of the egg whites. Don't overmix.

5. Bake for 15 minutes. Do the toothpick test to know if the muffins need more cooking time.

6. Let them cool and serve.

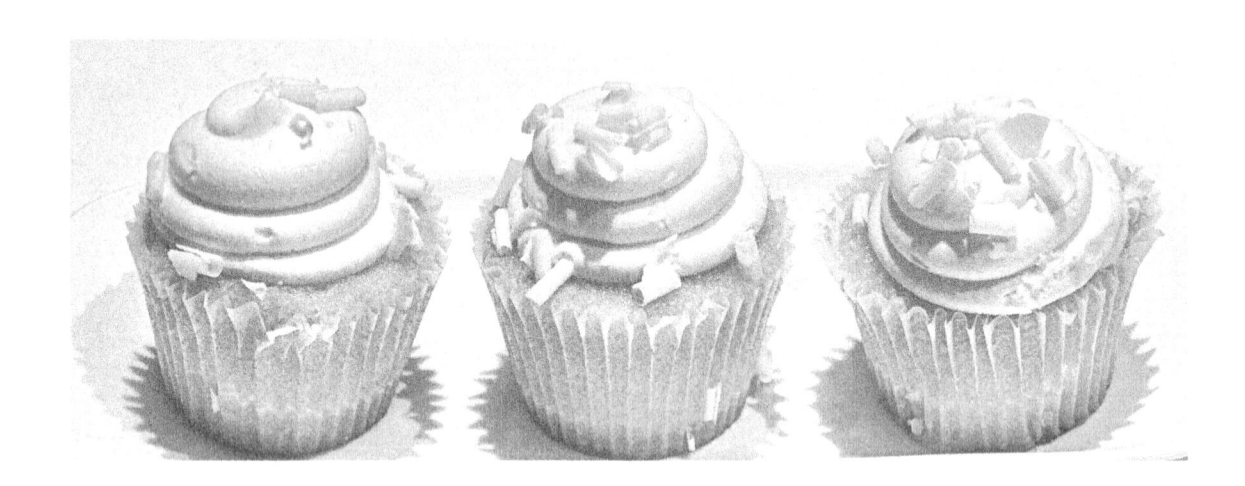

Blueberry & Cream Cheese Muffins

Yields: 12 muffins

Nutrition Facts: Amount per serving (1 muffin)

- ➤ Carbohydrates – 2g
- ➤ Protein – 3g
- ➤ Total Fat – 14g
- ➤ Calories – 155

Ingredients:

a. 16 oz. cream cheese, softened at room temperature
b. ½ cup Monkfruit sweetener
c. ¼ cup blueberries
d. ¼ cup almonds, sliced
e. ½ tsp. vanilla extract, sugar-free
f. ¼ tsp. xanthan gum
g. 2 eggs

Directions:

1. Preheat the oven to 350° F (180° C).
2. Beat the cream cheese until creamy and smooth.
3. Mix in the eggs, vanilla, sweetener, and xanthan gum. Beat until well-combined.

4. Fold in the almonds and blueberries.

5. Spoon the batter into a lined 12-piece muffin tin.

6. Bake for 20 minutes or more. Check if it's done using the toothpick test.

7. Cool at room temperature for a few minutes then refrigerate. They're best served when chilled.

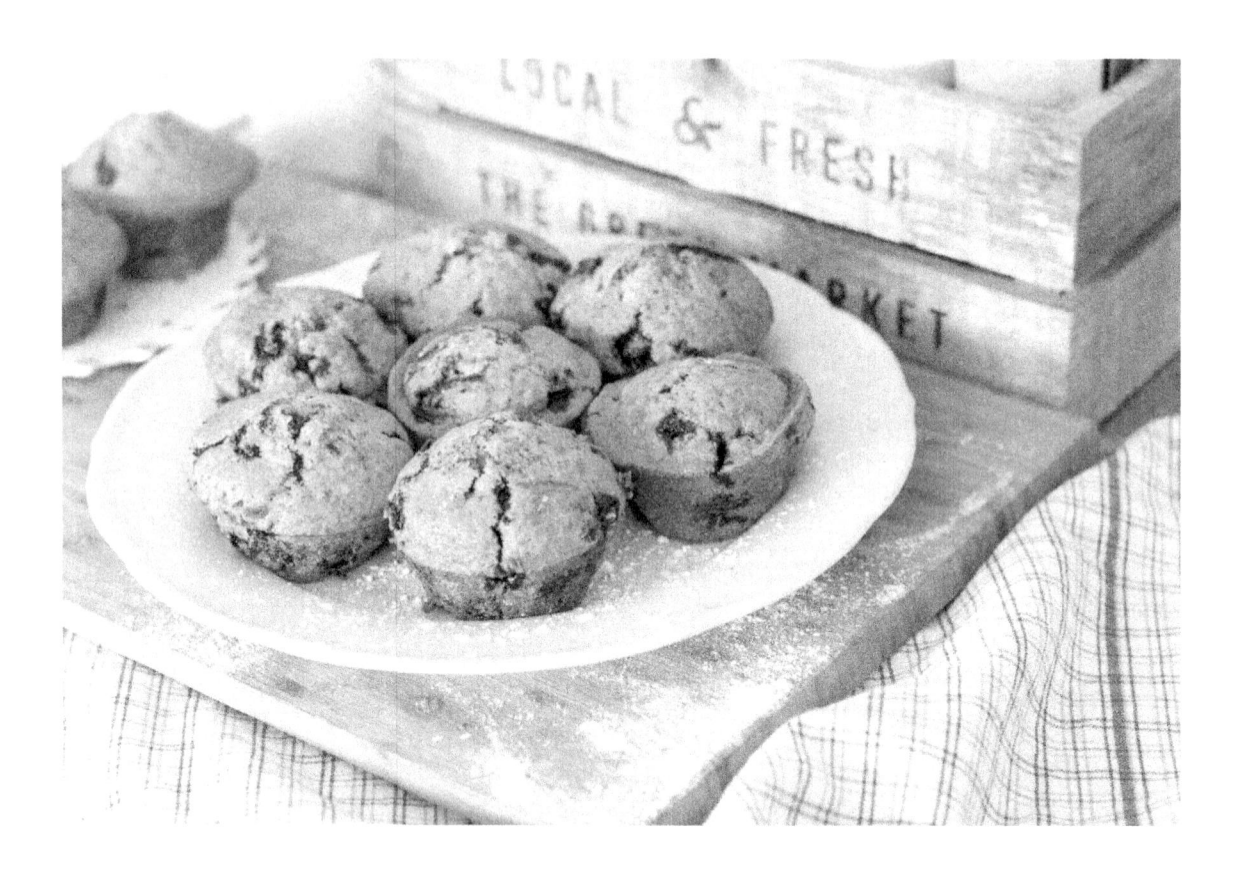

Chocolate Chip Muffins

Yields: 12 muffins

Nutrition Facts: Amount per serving (1 muffin)

- ➢ Carbohydrates – 9g
- ➢ Protein – 7g
- ➢ Total Fat – 26g
- ➢ Calories – 201

Ingredients:

a. 3 oz. butter, unsalted, melted
b. 1 cup almond flour
c. 2/3 cup heavy cream
d. ½ cup Erythritol sweetener
e. ½ cup cocoa powder, unsweetened
f. ½ cup chocolate chips, sugar-free
g. 1 ½ tsp. baking powder
h. 1 tsp. vanilla extract
i. 3 eggs

Directions:

1. Preheat the oven to 350° F (180° C) and line a 12-piece muffin tray.
2. Combine the Erythritol, cocoa powder, flour, and baking powder and mix well. Add the eggs, heavy cream, and vanilla. Mix until well-combined.
3. Stir in the chocolate chips and mix until well-combined.
4. Evenly scoop the mixture to the muffin tray.
5. Bake for about 20 minutes or until puffy. The muffins should spring back a bit when touched.
6. Cool a while and serve. The muffins may shrink a little when cooled.

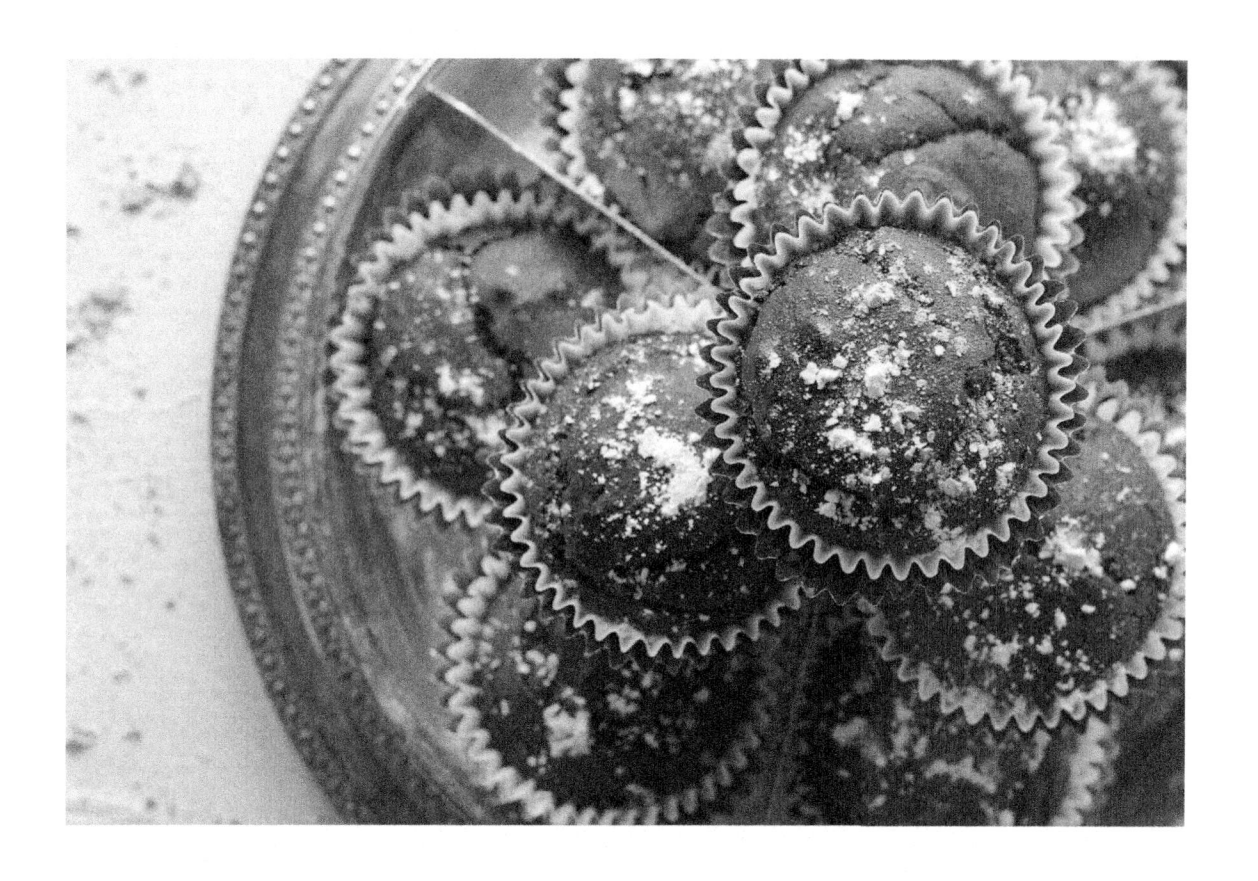

Strawberry Muffins with Coconut Cream Glaze

Yields: 12 muffins

Nutrition Facts: Amount per serving (1 muffin)

- Carbohydrates – 6g
- Protein – 7g
- Total Fat – 25g
- Calories – 257

Ingredients: (Muffin)

a. 3 cups almond flour
b. 2 cups strawberries, chopped
c. ¼ cup Erythritol sweetener
d. ½ cup ghee, melted
e. 1 tbsp. vanilla extract
f. 1 tbsp. lemon zest
g. 1 tsp. baking soda
h. 3 eggs, whisked

(Glaze)

a. 4 tbsp. coconut cream
b. 1 tbsp. Erythritol sweetener

Directions:

1. Preheat your oven to 350° F (180° C) and grease a 12-piece muffin tin.
2. In a large bowl, combine the muffin ingredients and mix well. Then, fold in the strawberries gently.
3. Pour the mixture in the muffin tins. Evenly divide the mixture.
4. Baker for about 16-18 minutes or more. Check if they're done by doing the toothpick test.
5. Remove from the oven and let them cool completely.
6. Combine the glaze ingredients and mix well. Let it sit at room temperature until thickened.
7. Drizzle the glaze over the muffins before serving.

Raspberry Muffins

Yields: 12 muffins

Nutrition Facts: Amount per serving (1 muffin)

- Carbohydrates – 3g
- Protein – 3g
- Total Fat – 8g
- Calories – 98

Ingredients: (Muffin)

a. 1 cup raspberries
b. 1 cup almond flour
c. 2/3 cup Erythritol sweetener
d. ¼ cup coconut flour
e. ¼ cup heavy cream
f. ¼ cup water
g. ¼ cup butter, melted
h. 2 tsp. baking powder
i. 1 tsp. almond extract
j. ¼ tsp. salt
k. 3 eggs, beaten

Directions:

1. Preheat your oven to 325° F (165° C) and line a 12-piece muffin tin.
2. Combine the flours, sweetener, salt, and baking powder. Set aside.
3. Whisk together the butter, water, heavy cream, extract, and eggs.
4. Add the wet mixture to the dry mixture. Mix together until well-combined. Then, fold in the raspberries gently.
5. Scoop the batter into the muffin tin. Each muffin would need ¼ cup of batter.
6. Bake for 35 minutes. Cool completely before serving.

Cranberry Muffins

Yields: 5 muffins

Nutrition Facts: Amount per serving (1 muffin)

- Carbohydrates – 5g
- Protein – 5g
- Total Fat – 13g
- Calories – 158

Ingredients: (Muffin)

a. 1/3 cup cranberries
b. ¼ cup coconut flour
c. ¼ cup unsalted butter, melted
d. 2 tbsp. heavy cream
e. 1 tsp. vanilla extract
f. 1 tsp. Stevia glycerite
g. ¼ tsp. sea salt
h. ¼ tsp. baking soda
i. 3 eggs, beaten

Directions:

1. Preheat your oven to 350° F (180° C). Prepare a muffin tin that fits 5 muffins and line with muffin liners.
2. Add the eggs, butter, vanilla, Stevia, salt, and milk in a bowl. Mix well, then add the coconut flour while continuing to stir until smooth.
3. Mix in the baking soda. Then, fold in the cranberries gently.
4. Scoop the batter into the muffin tin dividing it into portions evenly. You can top each muffin with extra cranberries.
5. Bake for 15 minutes or until it passes the toothpick test. Let them cool before removing from the tin and serving.

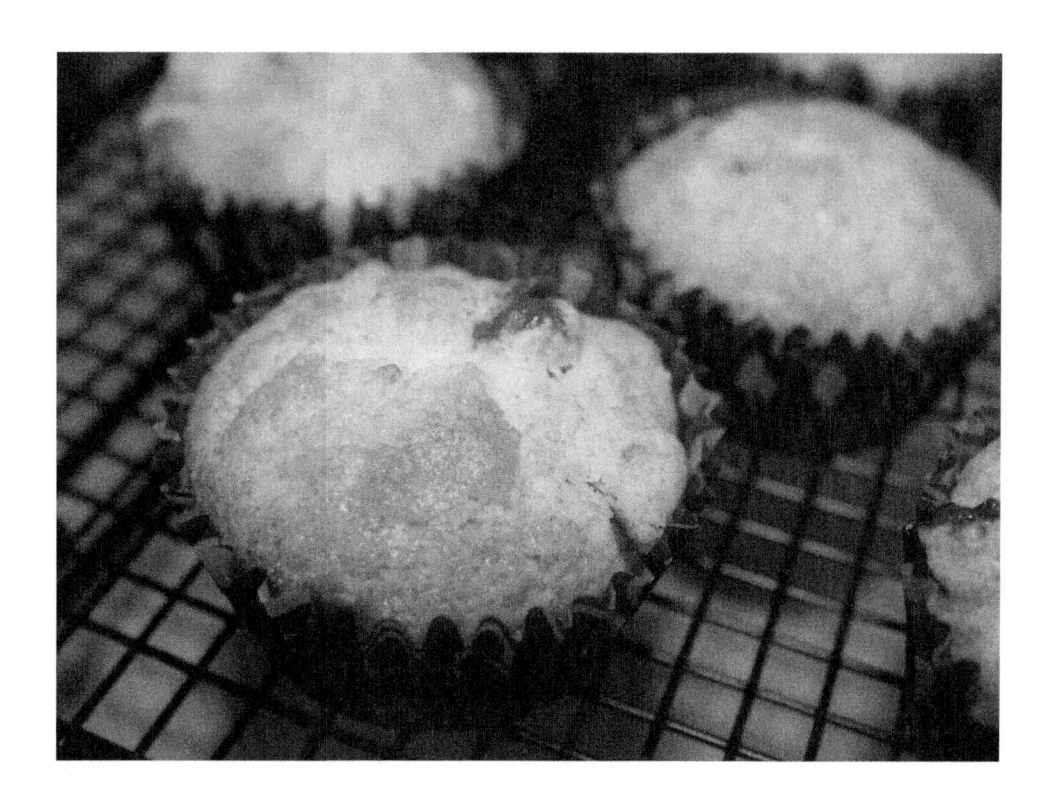

Easy Banana Muffins

Yields: 12 muffins

Nutrition Facts: Amount per serving (1 muffin)

- Carbohydrates – 5g
- Protein – 3g
- Total Fat – 8g
- Calories – 107

Ingredients: (Muffin)

a. 1 ¼ cup almond flour
b. 1 tbsp. coconut oil
c. ½ tsp. baking soda
d. 2-3 bananas, mashed
e. A pinch of salt
f. 1 egg

Directions:

1. Preheat your oven to 350° F (180° C). Line a 12-piece muffin tin.
2. Mix the eggs, coconut oil, and bananas well. Then, add the rest of the ingredients. Mix until well-combined.
3. Bake 20-25 minutes. Cool completely before serving.

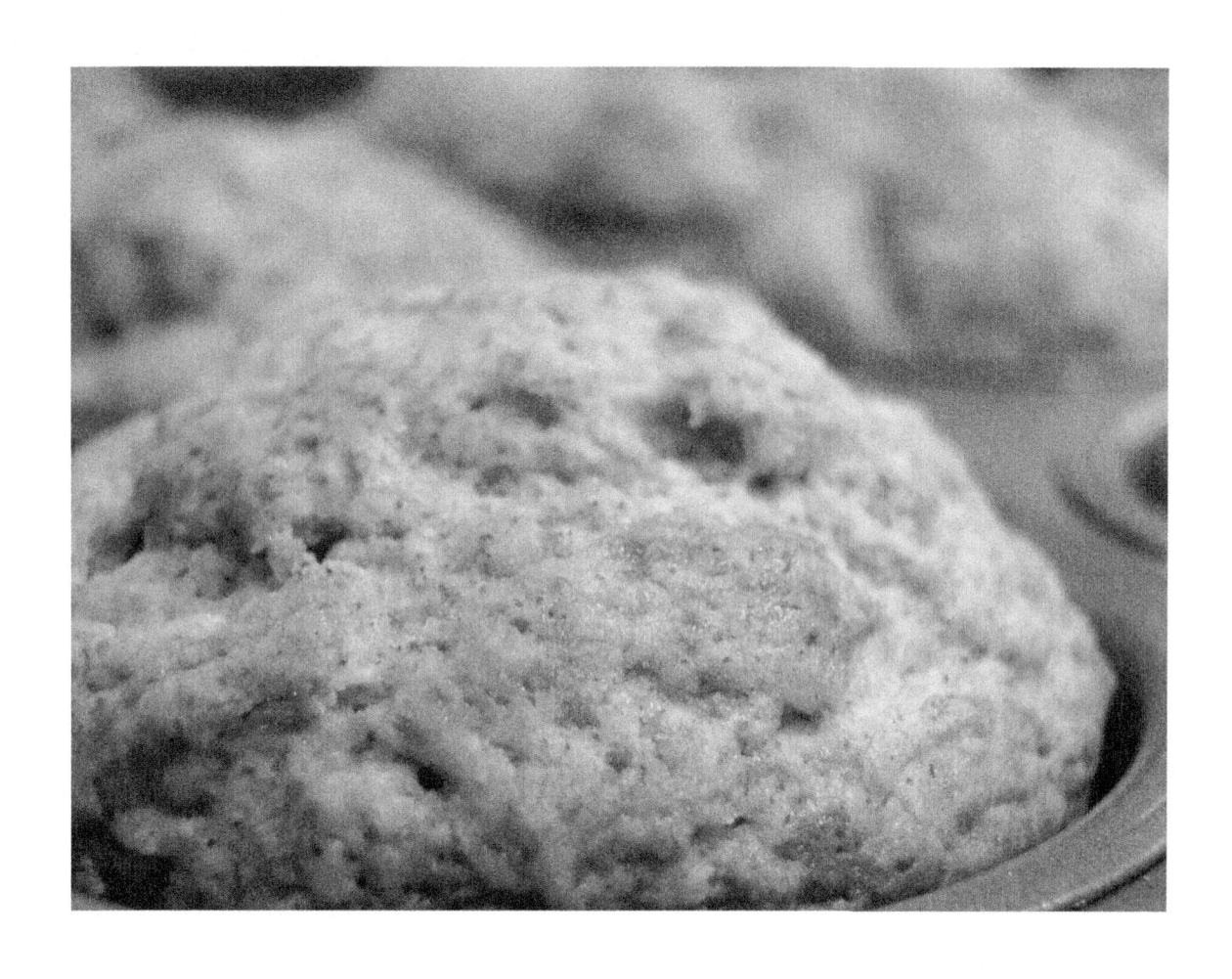

CHAPTER 6

Keto Crackers and Breadsticks

3-Ingredient Crackers

Yields: 6 servings

Nutrition Facts: Amount per serving (5 crackers)

- Carbohydrates – 8g
- Protein – 9g
- Total Fat – 19g
- Calories – 226

Ingredients:

a. 2 cups blanched almond flour
b. ½ tsp. sea salt
c. 1 large egg, beaten

Directions:

1. Prepare a baking sheet and line with parchment paper. Preheat your oven to 350° F (180° C).
2. Combine and flour and salt and mix well.

3. Mix in the egg. Continue to mix to form a dough.

4. Roll out and form into a rectangle with a thickness of 0.2cm

5. Cut the dough into 30 pieces. Prick the centers of each dough piece with a fork.

6. Place onto the baking sheet with spaces in between them.

7. Bake for about 8-12 minutes or until golden brown.

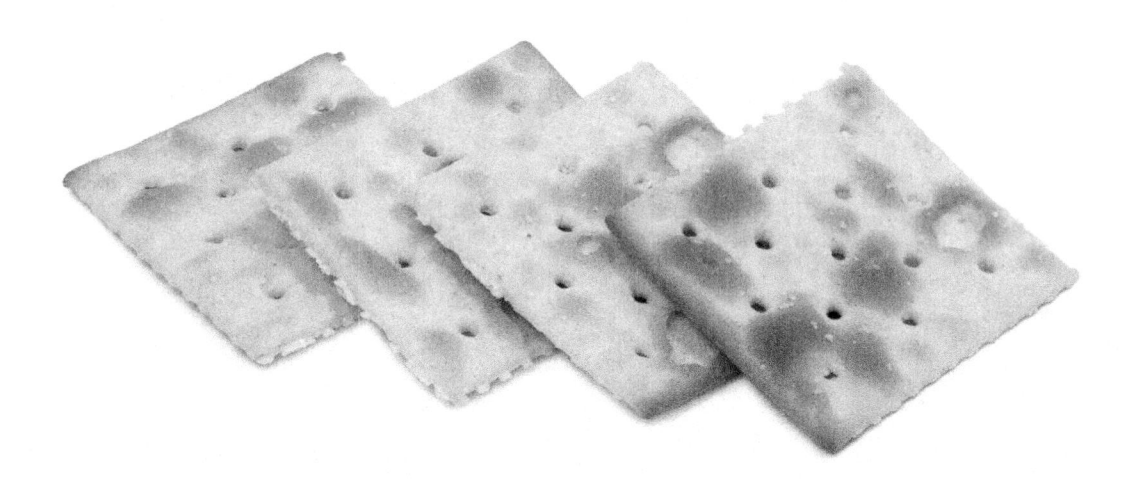

Rosemary & Flax Seed Crackers

Yields: Many

Nutrition Facts: Amount per serving (1 batch of the recipe)

- Carbohydrates – 34g
- Protein – 55g
- Total Fat – 70g
- Calories – 998

Ingredients:

a. 1 cup flax seeds, ground
b. ½ cup parmesan, grated
c. 1 tsp. rosemary, minced
d. Sea salt for sprinkling
e. 2 eggs

Directions:

1. Prepare a baking sheet and line with parchment paper. Preheat your oven to 350° F (180° C).
2. Combine and flour and salt and mix well.
3. Mix in the egg. Continue to mix to form a dough.
4. Roll out and form into a rectangle with a thickness of 0.2cm

5. Cut the dough into 30 pieces. Prick the centers of each dough piece with a fork.

6. Place onto the baking sheet with spaces in between them.

7. Bake for about 8-12 minutes or until golden brown.

Cheese & Basil Crackers

Yields: 24 pieces

Nutrition Facts: Amount per serving (1 piece)

- Carbohydrates – 0.9g
- Protein – 1.7g
- Total Fat – 5g
- Calories – 58

Ingredients:

a. 1 cup cheddar, coarsely grated

b. ¼ cup coconut flour

c. ¼ cup parmesan

d. 6 tbsp. butter, softened at room temperature

e. 2 tbsp. heavy whipping cream

f. 2 tbsp. basil, chopped

Directions:

1. Prepare 2 baking sheets lined with parchment paper. Preheat your oven to 325° F (165° C).
2. Put the butter and cream in a bowl and mix well.
3. Add the cheeses and combine. Then, add the flour. Mix them all well.

4. Add the basil and fold in gently. Make sure it's well-incorporated into the batter.

5. Roll out the dough until it's ¼-inch thick.

6. Create 24 crackers from the dough using a cooking cutter.

7. Place the crackers onto the baking sheet and bake for 12 minutes. Monitor the crackers so they don't burn.

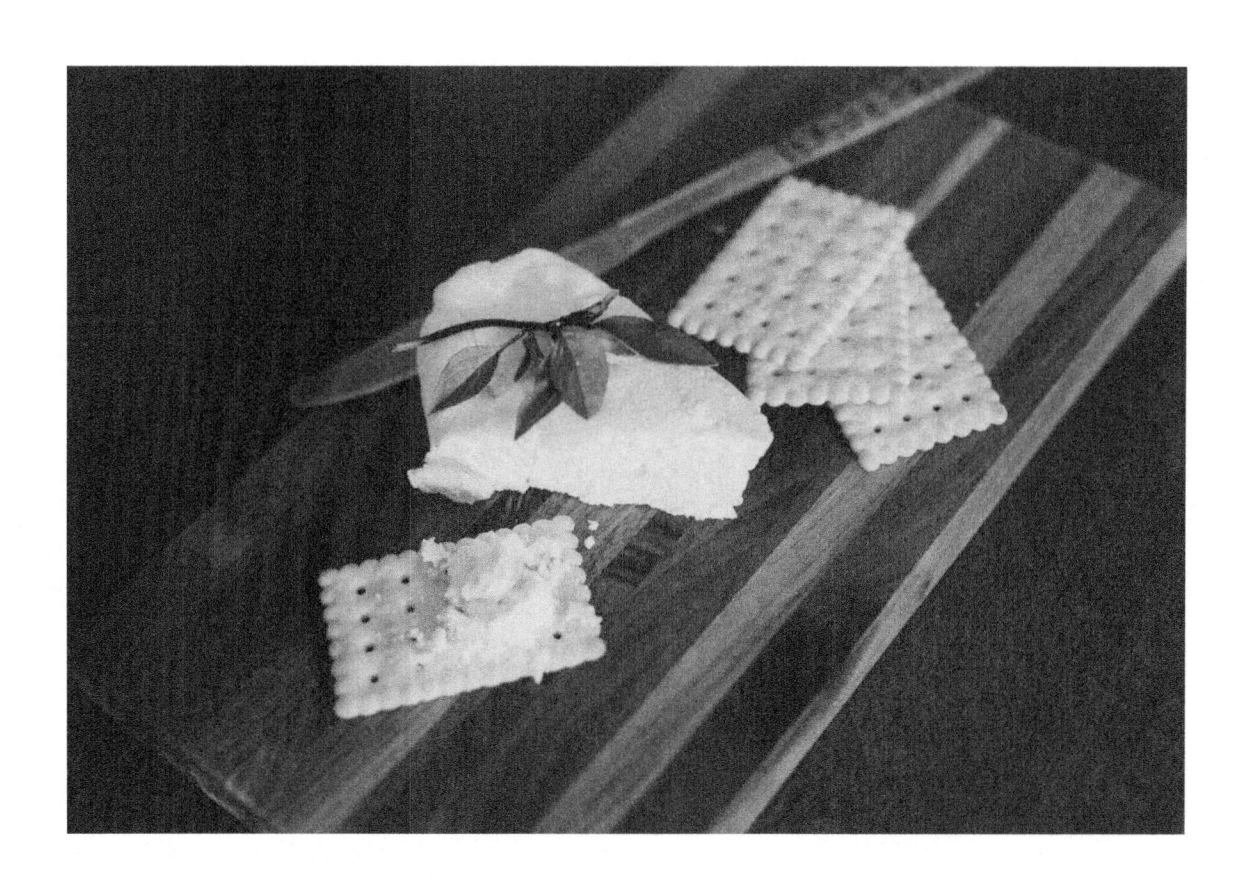

Almond & Coconut Crisps

Yields: 12 pieces

Nutrition Facts: Amount per serving (1 piece)

- Carbohydrates – 1.69g
- Protein – 10.68g
- Total Fat – 6g
- Calories – 64

Ingredients:

a. 1/3 cup Swerve Sweetener
b. ¼ cup butter
c. ¼ cup almond meal
d. 6 tbsp. shredded coconut
e. 2 tsp. yacon syrup
f. ¼ tsp. xanthan gum
g. ½ tsp. vanilla extract

Directions:

1. Preheat the oven to 350° F (180° C). Use parchment paper to line 2 baking sheets.
2. Cook the butter, syrup and Swerve over medium heat until dissolved and bubbly at the edges of the saucepan.

3. Remove from the heat and add the xanthan gum. Whisk vigorously.
4. Mix in the coconut, almond meal, and vanilla until well-combined.
5. Place the batter onto the baking sheet by a teaspoon. Leave 4-inch spaces between the crackers.
6. Wet your hands and slightly press down on the crackers.
7. Bake one baking sheet at a time. Place the sheet in the upper third of your oven. Bake for 8-12 minutes or until the edges become dark golden and spread out.
8. Cool the crackers completely before removing from the sheet or else they'll break.

Butter Crackers

Yields: 12 servings x 4 crackers

Nutrition Facts: Amount per serving (4 crackers)

- Carbohydrates – 2g
- Protein – 2g
- Total Fat – 8g
- Calories – 90

Ingredients:

a. 2 ¼ cups almond flour
b. 8 tbsp. salted butter, softened
c. Salt to taste
d. 2 egg whites

Directions:

1. Preheat the oven to 350° F (180° C). Line a large baking sheet (you can use several baking sheets).
2. Combine the flour and butter in a bowl and mix well. Add a dash of salt and the egg whites. Mix until you form a dough.
3. Roll the dough until it's 1/8-inch thick. Score your dough into 1 ½-inch squares. Sprinkle it with salt.

4. Bake for about 10-15 minutes until crackers become light brown.
5. Remove from the oven and cool. Gently break the crackers along the scores before serving.

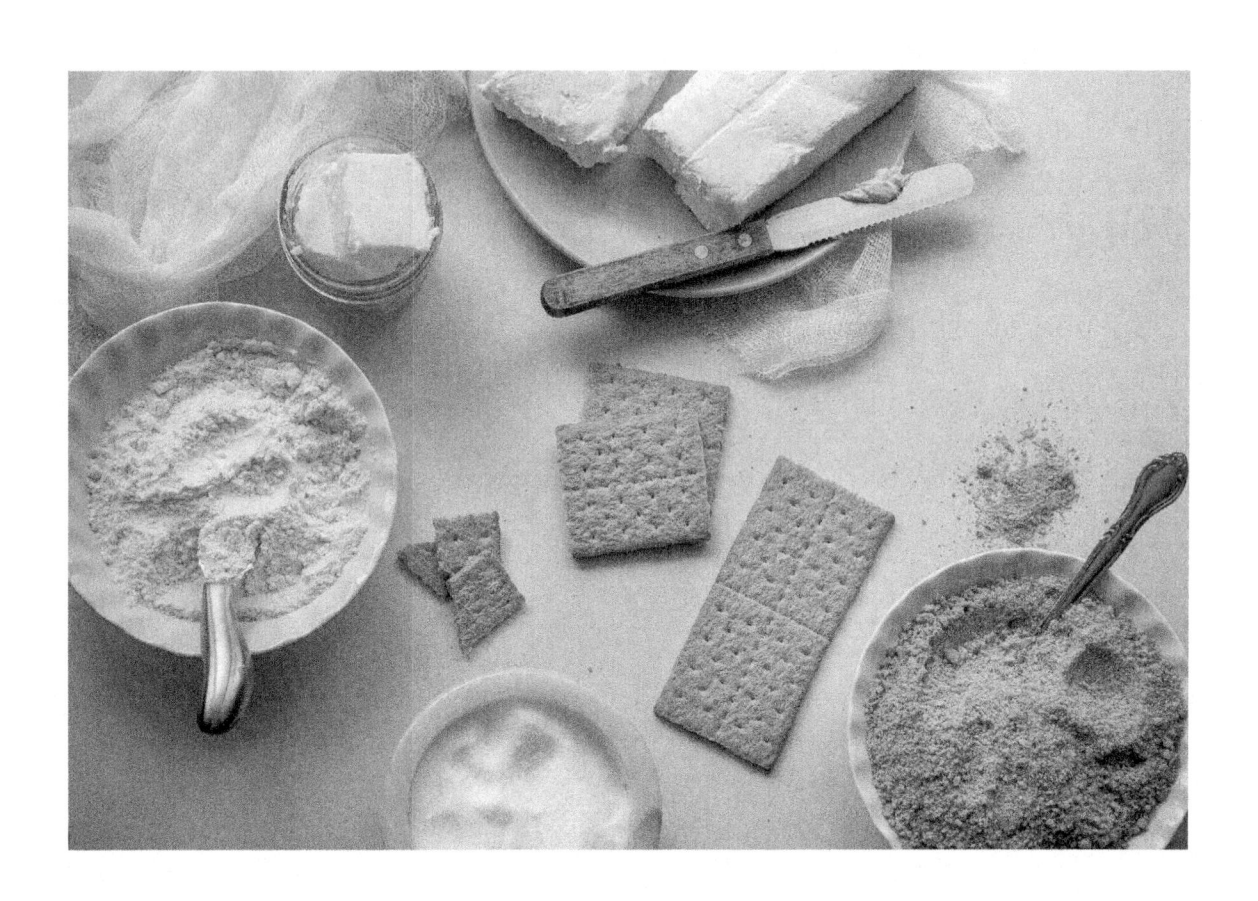

Thyme Crackers

Yields: Many

Nutrition Facts: Amount per serving (1 batch of the recipe)

- ➢ Carbohydrates – 6.8g
- ➢ Protein – 10g
- ➢ Total Fat – 22.6g
- ➢ Calories – 271

Ingredients:

a. 2 ½ cups almond flour
b. ½ cup coconut flour
c. 1 tbsp. extra-virgin olive oil
d. 1 tsp. flaxseed meal, ground
e. ½ tsp. onion powder
f. ½ tsp. dried thyme, chopped
g. ¼ tsp. kosher salt
h. 3 eggs

Directions:

1. Preheat your oven to 325° F (165° C) and line a baking sheet.
2. Mix in all the ingredients except for the eggs and oil in a bowl.

3. Then, add the oil and eggs. Mix well for a minute until you form a dough.
4. Roll out the dough until it's ¼-inch thick. Cut the dough into squares and transfer to the baking sheet.
5. Bake for 12-15 minute until golden brown.
6. Let the crackers cool before storing.

Herbed Crackers

Yields: Many

Nutrition Facts: Amount per serving (1 batch of the recipe)

- Carbohydrates – 12.9g
- Protein – 10.7g
- Total Fat – 22.7g
- Calories – 304

Ingredients:

a. All the ingredients for the **Thyme Crackers** recipe, but replace the onion powder and thyme with 1 tbsp. Italian seasoning

Directions:

1. Follow the directions for the **Thyme Crackers** recipe. Take note of the ingredient changes for this recipe.

Sour Cream & Chive Crackers

Yields: Many (40-80 crackers depending on size)

Nutrition Facts: Amount per serving (1 batch of the recipe)

- Carbohydrates – 6.8g
- Protein – 10g
- Total Fat – 22.6g
- Calories – 271

Ingredients:

a. 1.5 oz. sour cream, full-fat
b. 2 cups almond flour
c. 1 tsp. sea salt
d. ½ tsp. garlic powder
e. ½ cup chives, chopped

Directions:

1. Preheat the oven to 250° F (130° C) and line a baking sheet with parchment paper.
2. Mix all the ingredients by hand and knead until smooth.
3. Roll out the dough as thin as you can and transfer onto the baking sheet.
4. Cut into squares. The amount of crackers will depend on the sizes you cut.
5. Bake for 50-60 minutes. Monitor the crackers for they won't burn.

6. Cool and break the crackers with the slices you made.

Basic Breaksticks

Yields: 24 breadsticks

Nutrition Facts: Amount per serving (4 breadsticks)

- Carbohydrates – 12.8g
- Protein – 5.4g
- Total Fat – 18.8g
- Calories – 235.8

Ingredients:

a. 2 cups mozzarella, grated
b. 2/4 cup almond flour
c. 3 tbsp. cream cheese
d. 1 tbsp. psyllium husk powder
e. 1 tsp. baking powder
f. 1 large egg

Directions:

1. Preheat the oven to 400° F (200° C) line a baking sheet with parchment paper.
2. Add the cream cheese and egg in a bowl and combine slightly.
3. Combine all the dry ingredients except the mozzarella in a separate bowl.

4. Melt the mozzarella in the microwave with intervals until it's sizzling.
5. Add the cream cheese mixture and dry ingredients to the cheese. Mix well together.
6. Knead the dough. Then, press it flat on a silicone baking liner or parchment paper.
7. Cut the dough into 24 equal sticks. Only use a pizza cutter when using a silicone liner.
8. Transfer the breadsticks to a lined baking sheet. Place the baking sheet on the top rack of your oven. Bake for 13-15 minutes until crisp.

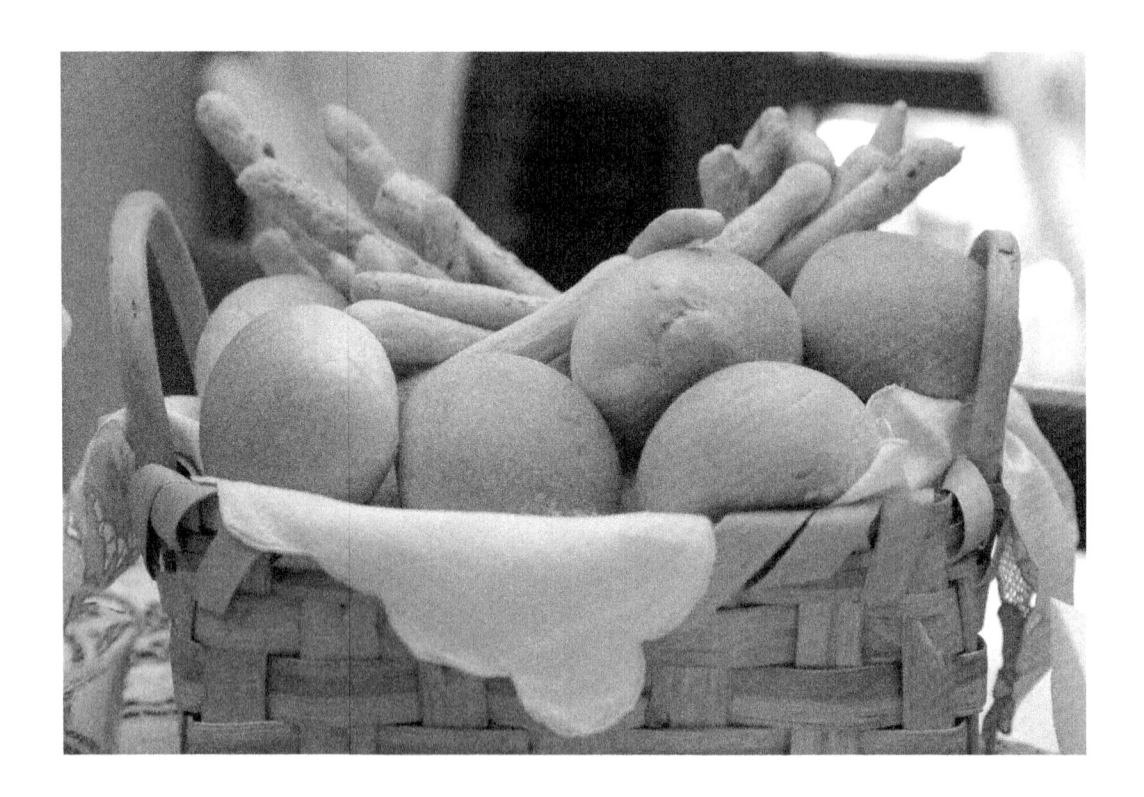

Cheesy Breaksticks

Yields: 24 breadsticks

Nutrition Facts: Amount per serving (4 breadsticks)

- Carbohydrates – 6.3g
- Protein – 18g
- Total Fat – 24.7g
- Calories – 314

Ingredients:

a. All the ingredients for the **Basic Breaksticks** recipe.
b. 3 oz. cheddar, grated
c. ¼ cup parmesan, grated
d. 1 tsp. garlic powder
e. 1 tsp. onion powder

Directions:

1. Follow the directions for the **Basic Breaksticks** recipe. Just include the additional ingredients for step 3.

Italian-Style Breaksticks

Yields: 24 breadsticks

Nutrition Facts: Amount per serving (4 breadsticks)

- Carbohydrates – 5.4g
- Protein – 12.8g
- Total Fat – 18.8g
- Calories – 237.7

Ingredients:

a. All the ingredients for the **Basic Breaksticks** recipe.

b. 2 tbsp. Italian seasoning

c. 1 tsp. salt

d. 1 tsp. pepper

Directions:

1. Follow the directions for the **Basic Breaksticks** recipe. Don't forget to include the additional ingredients for step 3.

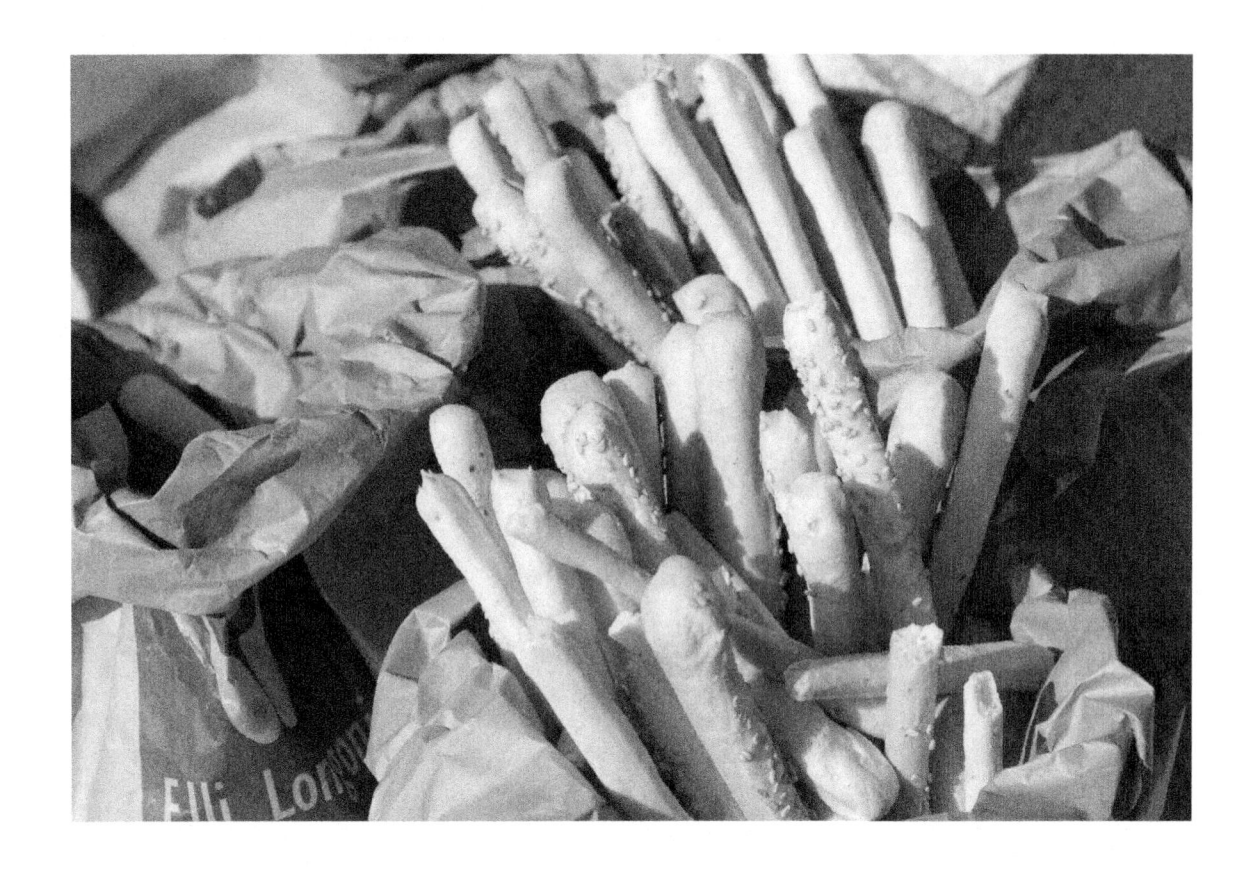

Cinnamon Breaksticks

Yields: 24 breadsticks

Nutrition Facts: Amount per serving (4 breadsticks)

- ➢ Carbohydrates – 7.1g
- ➢ Protein – 13g
- ➢ Total Fat – 24.3g
- ➢ Calories – 291.7

Ingredients:

a. All the ingredients for the **Basic Breaksticks** recipe.
b. 3 tbsp. Swerve sweetener
c. 3 tbsp. butter
d. 2 tbsp. cinnamon

Directions:

1. Follow the directions for the **Basic Breaksticks** recipe. Add the additional ingredients for step 3.

Easy Cheese & Garlic Breadsticks

Yields: 8 breadsticks

Nutrition Facts: Amount per serving (1 breadstick)

- Carbohydrates – 3g
- Protein – 7.3g
- Total Fat – 6.8g
- Calories – 102.6

Ingredients:

a. 1 cup mozzarella, low-moisture part-skim, grated
b. 1 cup parmesan, grated
c. 1 tsp. garlic powder
d. 1 egg

Directions:

1. Preheat the oven to 350° F (180° C) and prepare a lined baking sheet.
2. In a bowl, combine all the ingredients well.
3. Flatten the dough onto the lined baking sheet,
4. Bake for 15 minutes. Then, broil until the cheese melts and browns a little. Slice the bread into 8 sticks and serve

CHAPTER 7

Keto Cookies

Super Easy Peanut Butter Cookies

Yields: 8 cookies

Nutrition Facts: Amount per serving (1 cookie)

- Carbohydrates –2.1g
- Protein – 1.5g
- Total Fat –3.2g
- Calories – 41.6

Ingredients:

a. 1 cup peanut butter, sugar-free
b. ½ cup Stevia sweetener
c. 1 egg

Directions:

1. Preheat the oven to 350° F (180° C). Line a baking sheet with parchment paper.
2. Combine all the ingredients in a mixing bowl. Mix well.

3. Divide the batter into 8 and scoop onto the baking sheet. Using a fork, lightly press on the cookies.
4. Bake for 15 minutes or until golden brown.

Butter Cookies

Yields: 10 cookies

Nutrition Facts: Amount per serving (1 cookie)

- Carbohydrates –2g
- Protein – 2g
- Total Fat –10g
- Calories – 104

Ingredients:

a. 1 cup almond flour
b. ½ cup Erythritol sweetener
c. 4 tbsp. butter, softened
d. ½ tsp. vanilla extract

Directions:

1. Line a baking sheet with parchment paper. Preheat the oven to 350° F (180° C).
2. Mix all the ingredients in a mixing bowl until you form a dough.
3. Divide into 10 pieces and roll into balls. Place the balls onto the baking sheet with spaces in between.
4. Press on the dough balls with a fork lightly.
5. Bake for 10 minutes and let it cool before serving.

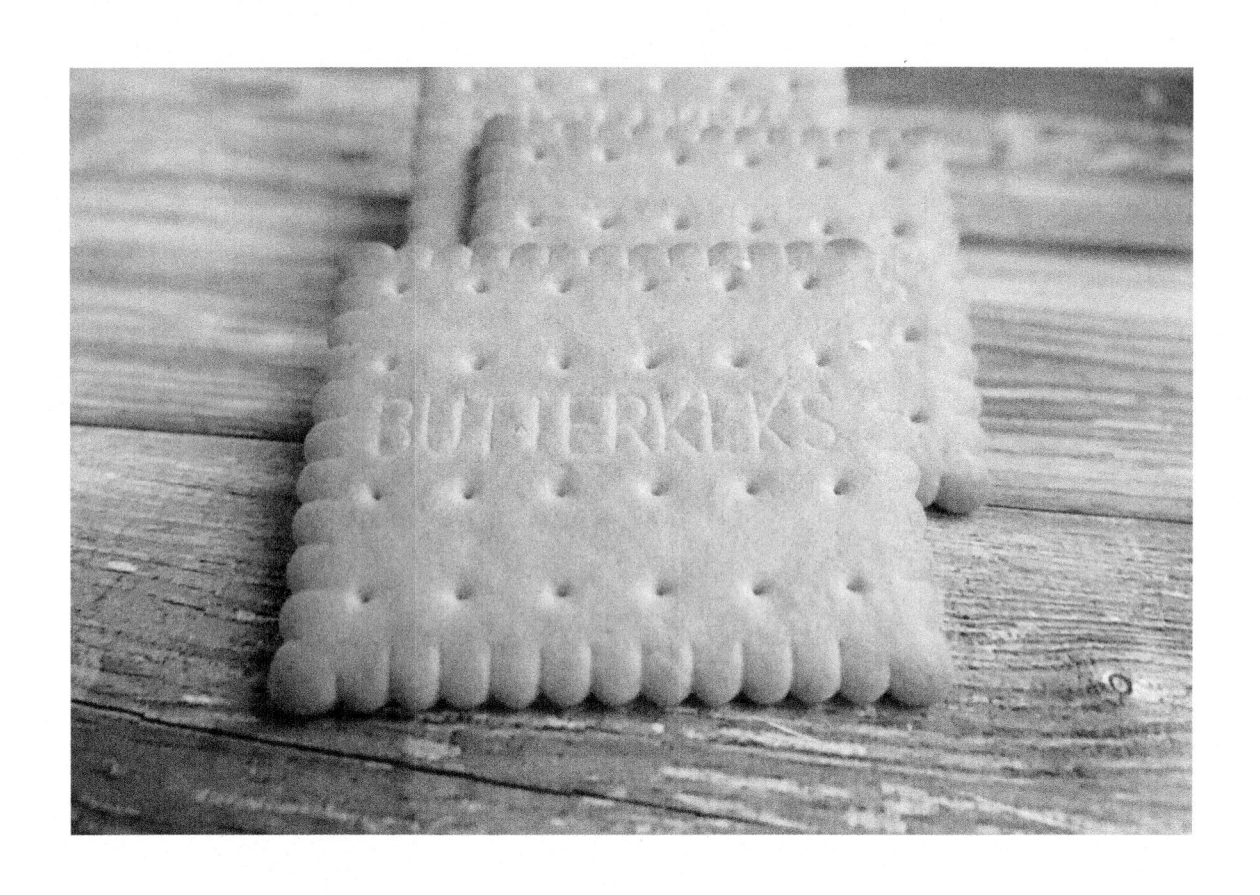

Cream Cheese Cookies

Yields: 24 cookies

Nutrition Facts: Amount per serving (1 cookie)

- ➢ Carbohydrates –3g
- ➢ Protein – 3g
- ➢ Total Fat –9g
- ➢ Calories – 106

Ingredients:

a. 2 oz. cream cheese, softened
b. 3 cups blanched almond flour
c. ½ cup Erythritol sweetener
d. ¼ cup butter, softened
e. 2 tsp. vanilla extract
f. ¼ tsp. sea salt
g. 1 large egg white

Directions:

1. Preheat the oven to 350° F (180° C). Prepare a lined baking sheet.
2. Mix the cream cheese, Erythritol, and butter until fluffy.

3. Add the salt, egg white, and vanilla. Beat and combine well. Then, mix in the flour half a cup at a time.

4. Scoop about 1 ½ tbsp. of the dough onto the baking sheet. You should get about 24 balls. Then, flatten the balls with your palm.

5. Bake for 15 minutes or until the edges turn lightly golden.

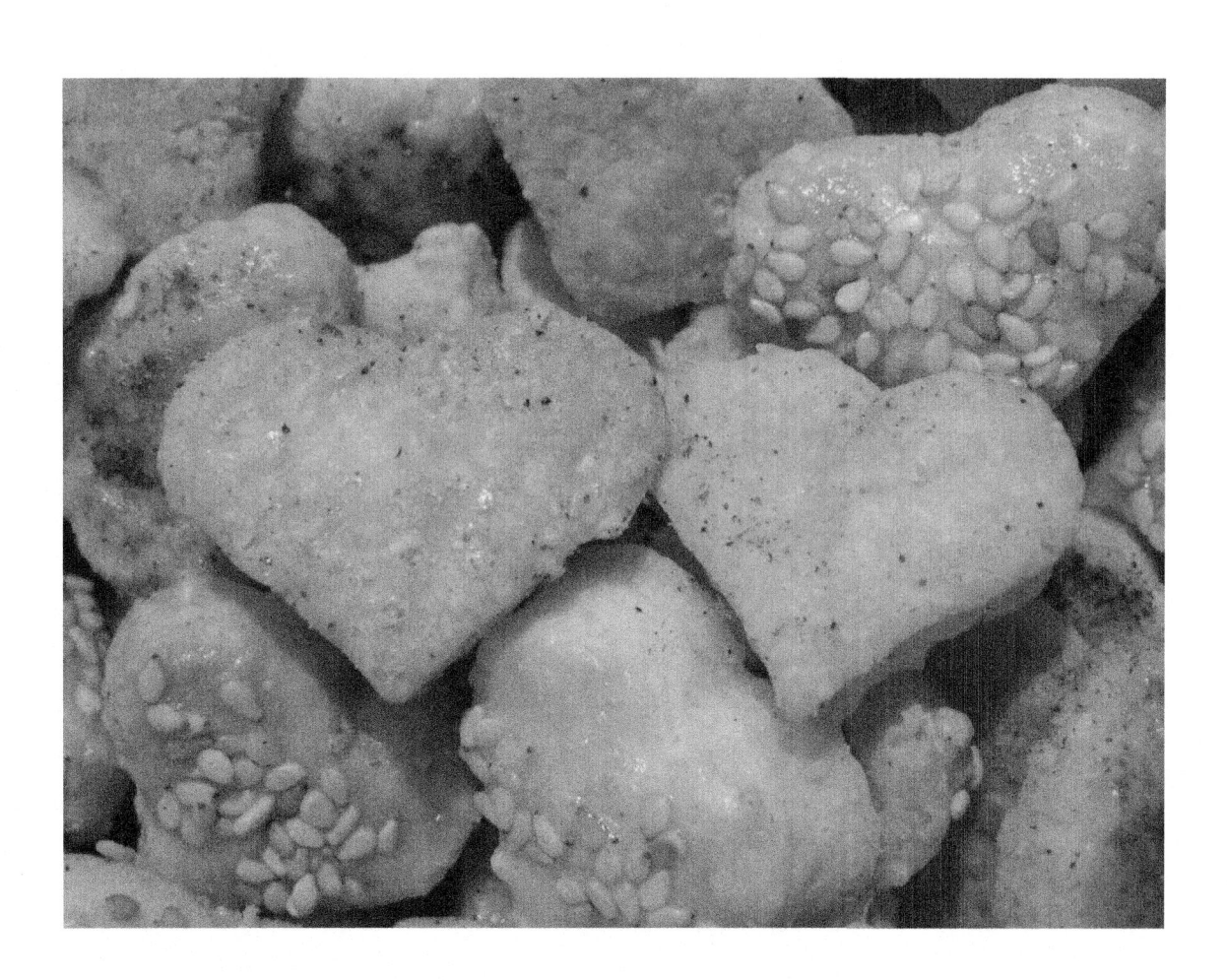

Macadamia Cookies

Yields: 24 cookies

Nutrition Facts: Amount per serving (1 cookie)

- Carbohydrates –3g
- Protein – 2g
- Total Fat –13g
- Calories – 132

Ingredients:

a. 12 oz. macadamia butter

b. ½ cup almond meal

c. 1/3 cup Xylitol sweetener

d. 1 tsp. cinnamon

e. 1 tsp. vanilla extract

f. 2 eggs

Directions:

1. Preheat the oven to 350° F (180° C).

2. Combine all the ingredients in a mixing bowl. Mix well until well-incorporated.

3. Create teaspoon-sized balls with the mixture. You should get 24 pieces.

4. Place the balls onto a lined baking sheet then press into desired size.

5. Bake for 12 minutes or until golden brown and edges harden.

Brownie Cookies

Yields: 14 cookies

Nutrition Facts: Amount per serving (1 cookie)

- Carbohydrates –2.9g
- Protein – 5.5g
- Total Fat –12.1g
- Calories – 141

Ingredients:

a. 1 cup almond butter, smoothened

b. ½ cup Erythritol sweetener

c. ¼ cup dark chocolate chips, sugar-free

d. 4 tbsp. cocoa powder, unsweetened

e. 3 tbsp. almond milk

f. 1 large egg

Directions:

1. Preheat the oven to 350° F (180° C).
2. Combine the butter, cocoa, sweetener, and egg. Mix well. Add in the almond milk and mix until soft and fudgy.
3. Fold in the chocolate chips carefully.

4. Make 14 balls with the batter. Place them on a lined baking sheet and press with your palm. It should be 1-cm thick.
5. Bake for 10-12 minutes or until little cracks form on the tops. Cool the cookies before serving to firm up.

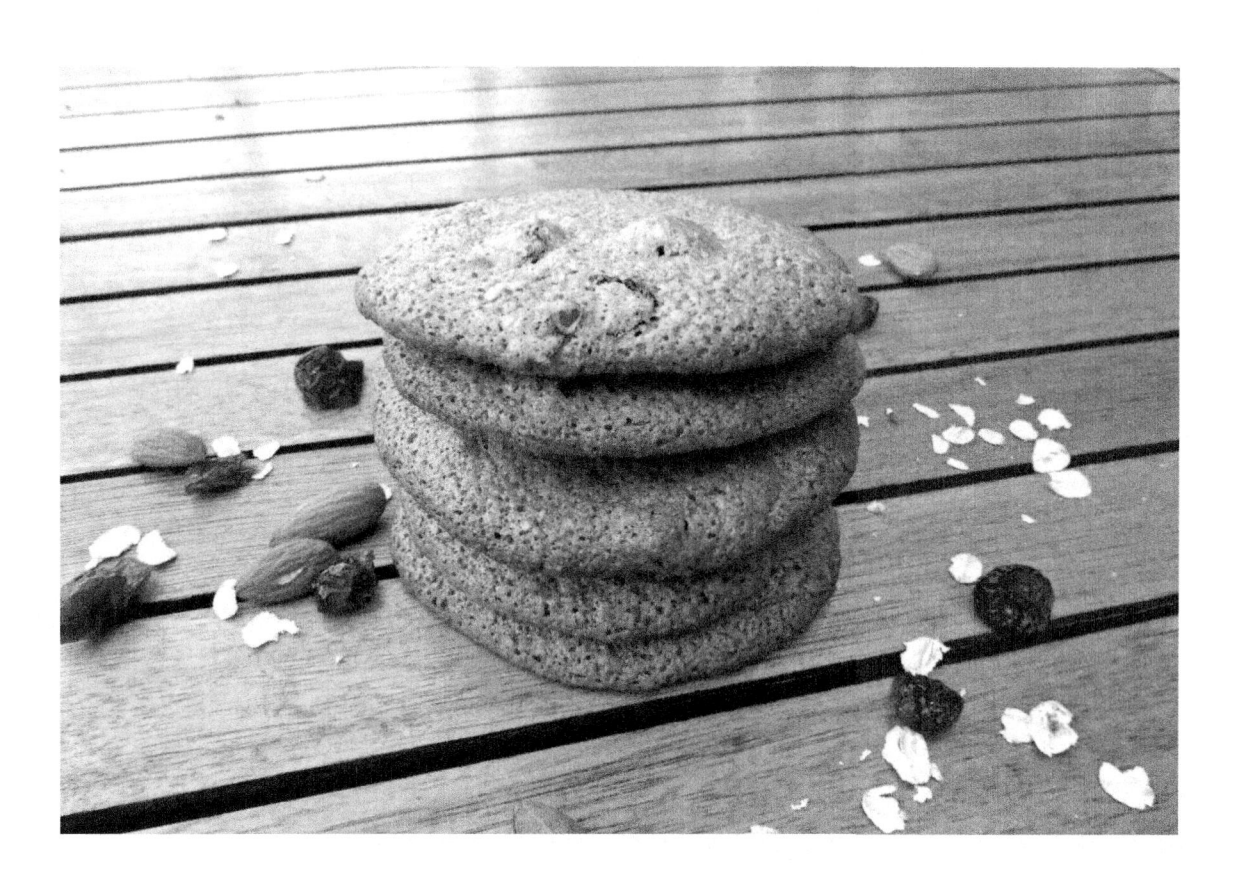

Basic Sugar Cookies

Yields: 10 cookies

Nutrition Facts: Amount per serving (1 cookie)

- Carbohydrates –5.1g
- Protein – 1.2g
- Total Fat –22.8g
- Calories – 210.9

Ingredients:

a. 1 cup extra-virgin olive oil
b. 1 cup Erythritol sweetener
c. ¼ cup oat fiber
d. ¼ cup coconut flour
e. ¼ cup almond flour
f. ¼ cup flax meal
g. ¼ cup water
h. 1 tbsp. vanilla extract
i. 1 tsp. baking powder
j. ¾ tsp. cider vinegar
k. 1/8 tsp. salt
l. 2 large eggs

Directions:

1. Preheat the oven to 350° F (180° C). Line a baking sheet with parchment paper.
2. Combine the oat fiber, coconut and almond flours, and flax meal. Mix well, then add in all the other ingredients. Knead until you get a dough that's slightly sticky.
3. Roll out the dough until it's ¼-inch thick. Cut the dough with a cookie cutter and place the cookies on the baking sheet. Sprinkle extra Erythritol on top.
4. Bake for 8-12 minutes or until done.

Lemon Sugar Cookies

Yields: 10 cookies

Nutrition Facts: Amount per serving (1 cookie)

- Carbohydrates –7.8g
- Protein – 1.3g
- Total Fat –23.7g
- Calories – 211.7

Ingredients:

a. All the ingredients for the **Basic Sugar Cookies** recipe
b. 1-2 cups Erythitol sweetener
c. 6-8 lemons, zested and juiced

Directions:

1. Follow the directions for the **Basic Sugar Cookies** recipe. But, add the lemon zest to the dough.
2. Let the cookies cool.
3. Mix the lemon juice and sweetener together. Adjust the amounts as necessary. You should get a slightly thick mixture.
4. Once the cookies are cooled, spread the icing over the cookies. Refrigerate or freeze to set the icing before serving.

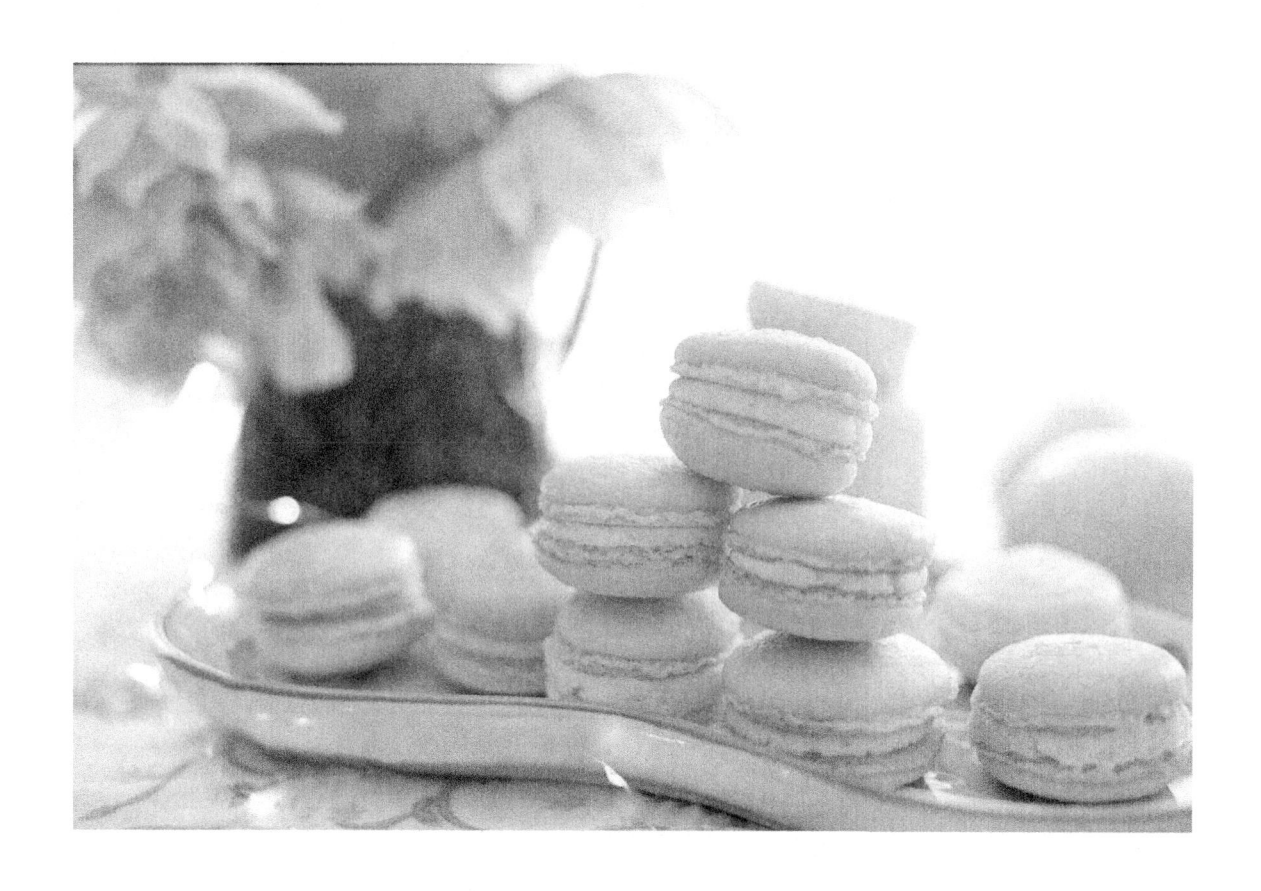

Chocolate Chip Cookies

Yields: 10 cookies

Nutrition Facts: Amount per serving (1 cookie)

- Carbohydrates –17.8g
- Protein – 2.1g
- Total Fat –29g
- Calories – 293.4

Ingredients:

a. All the ingredients for the **Basic Sugar Cookies** recipe
b. 1 cup dark chocolate chips, sugar-free

Directions:

1. Follow the directions for the **Basic Sugar Cookies** recipe.
2. But, before rolling out the cookie dough, fold in the chocolate chips.

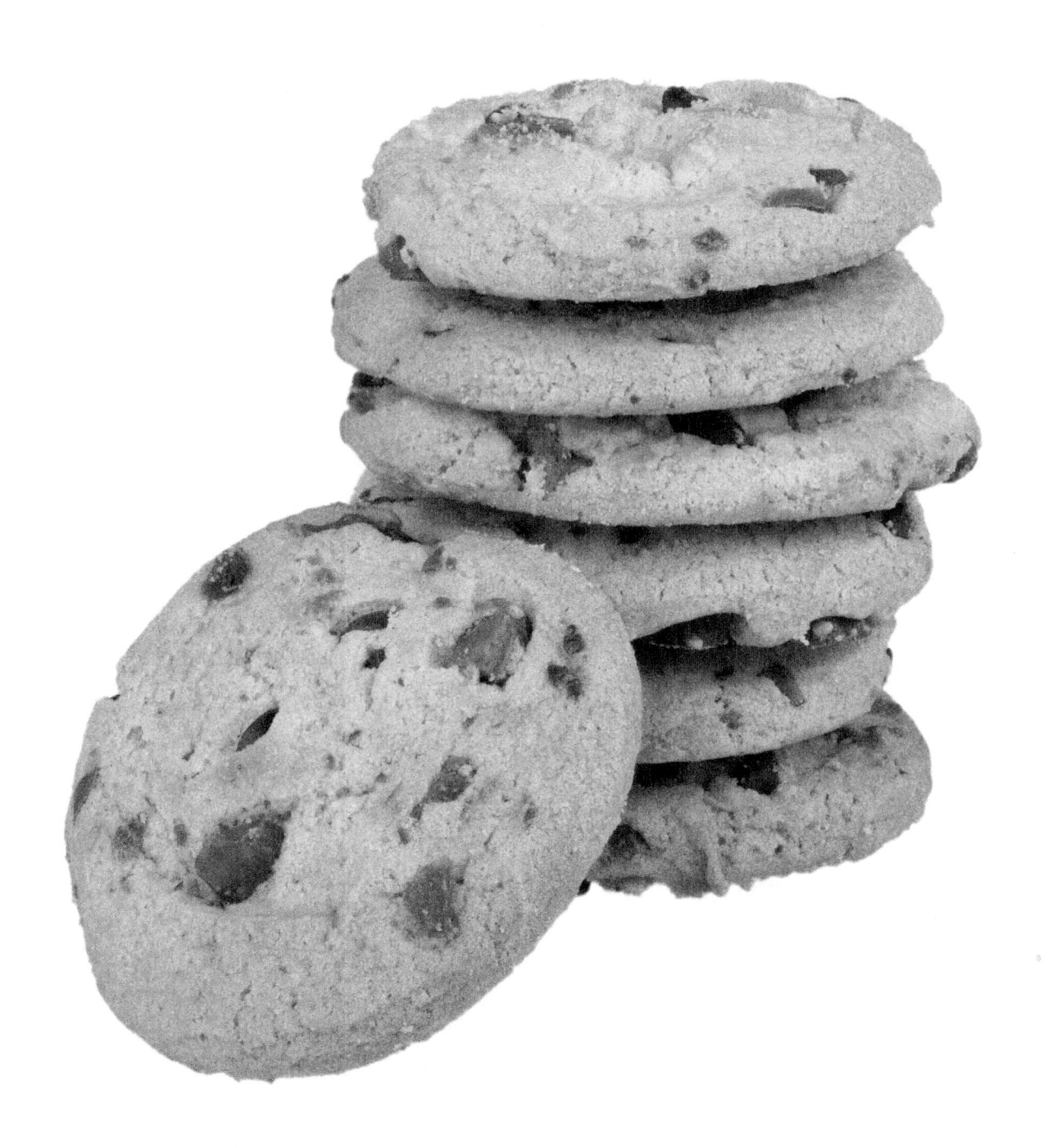

Walnut Cookies

Yields: 16 cookies

Nutrition Facts: Amount per serving (1 cookie)

- ➢ Carbohydrates –2g
- ➢ Protein – 1.5g
- ➢ Total Fat –11g
- ➢ Calories – 108

Ingredients:

a. 1 cup walnuts, ground
b. ½ cup Erythritol sweetener
c. ¼ cup coconut flour
d. 8 tbsp. butter, softened
e. 1 tsp. vanilla extract
f. 1 tsp. nutmeg ground

Directions:

1. Preheat the oven to 325° F (165° C). Prepare two baking sheets and line with parchment paper.

2. Mix all the ingredients together except for the butter. Once combined, mix in the butter until your form a soft dough.
3. Divide the dough into 16 and form into balls.
4. Place the balls onto the baking sheet and flatten.
5. Bake for 13 minutes. Let the cookies cool to firm up.

Raspberry Cookies

Yields: 10 cookies

Nutrition Facts: Amount per serving (1 cookie)

- Carbohydrates –13g
- Protein – 3g
- Total Fat –8g
- Calories – 132

Ingredients:

a. 4 oz. raspberries, chopped
b. 1 ¼ cups almond flour
c. ¼ cup coconut flour
d. ½ cup Erythritol sweetener
e. 1 tbsp. ghee, melted
f. 1 tsp. vanilla extract
g. 1 tsp. baking powder
h. 1 medium egg

Directions:

1. Preheat the oven to 350° F (180° C).
2. Mix the flours, Erythritol, and baking powder until well-combined. Then, mix in the raspberries. Combine well.

3. Whip the vanilla and egg together. Slowly add the ghee while continuing to whisk.

4. Add the wet mixture to the bowl of the dry mixture and mix until you form a dough.

5. Divide into 10 and roll into balls. Place on a lined baking sheet and flatten with your palm.

6. Bake for 10-12 minutes. Rotate the tray halfway through baking. Let the cookies cool before serving

Flourless Chocolate Chip Cookies

Yields: 18 cookies

Nutrition Facts: Amount per serving (1 cookie)

- Carbohydrates –8.6g
- Protein – 2.7g
- Total Fat –13.9g
- Calories – 147

Ingredients:

a. 1 cup dark chocolate chips, sugar-free
b. 1 cup coconut flakes
c. ¾ cup walnuts, chopped
d. ¼ cup coconut oil
e. 4 tbsp. butter, softened
f. 2 tbsp. Swerve sweetener
g. 4 egg yolks

Directions:

1. Preheat the oven to 350° F (180° C). Line a baking sheet with parchment paper.
2. Add the oil, butter, egg yolks, and Swerve in a large bowl. Mix together well. Then, add the chocolate chips, walnuts, and coconut.
3. Put a spoonful of the batter on the baking sheet. Repeat until everything is in the sheet. You should get 18 pieces.
4. Bake for 15 minutes or until the cookies turn golden brown.

Choco Fudge Cookies

Yields: 10 cookies

Nutrition Facts: Amount per serving (1 cookie)

- Carbohydrates –4.8g
- Protein – 4.4g
- Total Fat –11.6g
- Calories – 132

Ingredients:

a. 1 cup almond flour
b. ½ cup Swerve sweetener
c. ½ cup cocoa powder, unsweetened
d. ¼ cup butter
e. 1 tsp. vanilla extract
f. 1 tsp. baking powder
g. A pinch of sea salt
h. 2 eggs

Directions:

1. Preheat the oven to 350° F (180° C) and grease a baking sheet.
2. Combine the cocoa powder, butter, and Swerve and mix until well-combined.

3. Add the eggs, baking powder, and vanilla. Continue to mix well.

4. Lastly, add in the flour. Mix well until you get a thick batter.

5. Divide the batter into 10 and form into cookies. They don't expand much, so shape them as desired.

6. Bake for 12-15 minutes. Let them cool before serving.

CHAPTER 8

Keto Bread for Breakfast, Lunch, and Dinner

Quick Microwaveable Bread

Yields: 1 serving

Nutrition Facts: Amount per serving (1 serving)

- ➢ Carbohydrates –4g
- ➢ Protein – 4g
- ➢ Total Fat –21g
- ➢ Calories – 220

Ingredients:

- a. 3 tbsp. almond flour
- b. 1 tbsp. butter, melt
- c. ½ tsp. baking powder, double-acting
- d. 1 large egg

Directions:

1. Mix all the ingredients in a ramekin. Beat until well-combined.
2. Cook in the microwave for 90 seconds. Then, flip the bread on a plate and slice it in half. Toast in a toaster.
3. You can also bake for 10-12 minutes at 325° F (165° C).

Avocado Bacon Breakfast Muffins

Yields: 2 servings (15 muffins)

Nutrition Facts: Amount per serving (1 serving)

- ➢ Carbohydrates –8g
- ➢ Protein – 24g
- ➢ Total Fat –34g
- ➢ Calories – 380

Ingredients:

a. 1 can (13.5 oz.) coconut milk, unsweetened
b. ½ cup + 1 tsp. cheddar, grated
c. ½ cup almond meal
d. ¼ cup flax seed meal
e. 5 tbsp. butter, melted
f. 1 ½ tbsp. psyllium husk powder
g. 1 tbsp. lemon juice
h. 1 tsp. baking powder
i. 1 tsp. each of salt and pepper
j. ¼ tsp. each or red pepper flakes and garlic powder
k. 2 avocados, cubed
l. 1 green onion stalk, chopped
m. 5 bacon slices, cooked and chopped

n. 5 large eggs

Directions:

1. Preheat the oven to 350° F (180° C). Grease a 15-piece muffin tin or line with baking cups.
2. Mix all the ingredients together except for the avocado. Mix until well-combined.
3. Fold the avocado in the mixture carefully.
4. Bake for 25-30 minutes and cool before serving.

English Muffins

Yields: 3 servings

Nutrition Facts: Amount per serving (1 serving)

- Carbohydrates –4g
- Protein – 5g
- Total Fat –15g
- Calories – 159

Ingredients:

a. 3 tbsp. butter for frying
b. 2 tbsp. coconut flour
c. ½ tsp. baking powder
d. A dash of salt
e. 2 large eggs

Directions:

1. Mix the dry ingredients first and combine well.
2. Add in the eggs and whisk everything together. Leave for a few minutes.

3. Divide the batter into 3. Then, heat the butter in a pan over medium-high heat.
4. Fry each portion in the pan. Cook each side of the breads for a few minutes.

Blueberry Bread Loaf

Yields: 1 loaf (12 slices)

Nutrition Facts: Amount per serving (1 slice)

- ➢ Carbohydrates –4g
- ➢ Protein – 5g
- ➢ Total Fat –13g
- ➢ Calories – 156

Ingredients:

a. ½ cup almond flour
b. ½ cup almond butter, melted
c. ½ cup almond milk, unsweetened
d. ½ cup blueberries
e. ¼ cup ghee, melted
f. 2 tbsp. baking powder
g. ½ tsp. salt
h. 5 eggs, beaten

Directions:

1. Preheat your oven to 350° F (180° C). Line a loaf tin with parchment paper and grease lightly.
2. Combine the flour, baking powder, and salt in a bowl. Add the ghee and almond butter. Mix until well-combined.
3. Whisk the eggs and milk together before adding to the bowl. Mix well,
4. Fold in the blueberries into the batter and pour into the loaf tin.
5. Bake for 45 minutes or until it passes the toothpick test.
6. Completely cool the bread before removing from the tin.
7. To serve, slice the bread into 12 and toast each slice.

Broccoli & Cheddar Breakfast Bread

Yields: 1 loaf (10 slices)

Nutrition Facts: Amount per serving (1 slice)

- ➢ Carbohydrates –2.9g
- ➢ Protein – 6.6g
- ➢ Total Fat –5.1g
- ➢ Calories – 82.5

Ingredients:

a. 1 cup cheddar, grated
b. ¾ cup broccoli florets, raw, chopped
c. 4 tbsp. coconut flour
d. 2 tsp. baking powder
e. 1 tsp. salt
f. 5 eggs, beaten

Directions:

1. Grease and line a loaf tin. Preheat your oven to 350° F (180° C).
2. Combine all the ingredients and mix well

3. Pour the batter into the loaf tin.
4. Bake for 25-32 minutes or until golden brown and completely cooked.

Cloud Bread

Yields: 10 pieces

Nutrition Facts: Amount per serving (1 piece)

- Carbohydrates –0.9g
- Protein – 2.9g
- Total Fat – 3.8g
- Calories – 49.9

Ingredients:

a. 2 oz. cream cheese
b. 1 tsp. Italian seasoning
c. ½ tsp. cream of tartar
d. ½ tsp. sea salt
e. ¼ tsp. garlic powder
f. 4 large eggs, yolks and whites separated

Directions:

1. Preheat your oven to 300° F (150° C). Prepare 2 large baking sheets and line with parchment paper.
2. Whisk the egg whites with cream of tartar. Continue to whisk until stiff peaks form.

3. In a separate bowl, beat the cream cheese. Then, add the yolks one at a time. Continue to mix until smooth. Then, add the seasoning, garlic powder, and salt.

4. Fold the egg whites into the yolk mixture. Continue to fold to until foamy and firm.

5. Place ¼-cup portions of the batter onto the baking sheets. You should get 10 portions. Spread each into 4-inch rounds that's ¾-inch high.

6. Bake for 30 minutes or until golden and firm. Cool them completely before removing from the baking sheet.

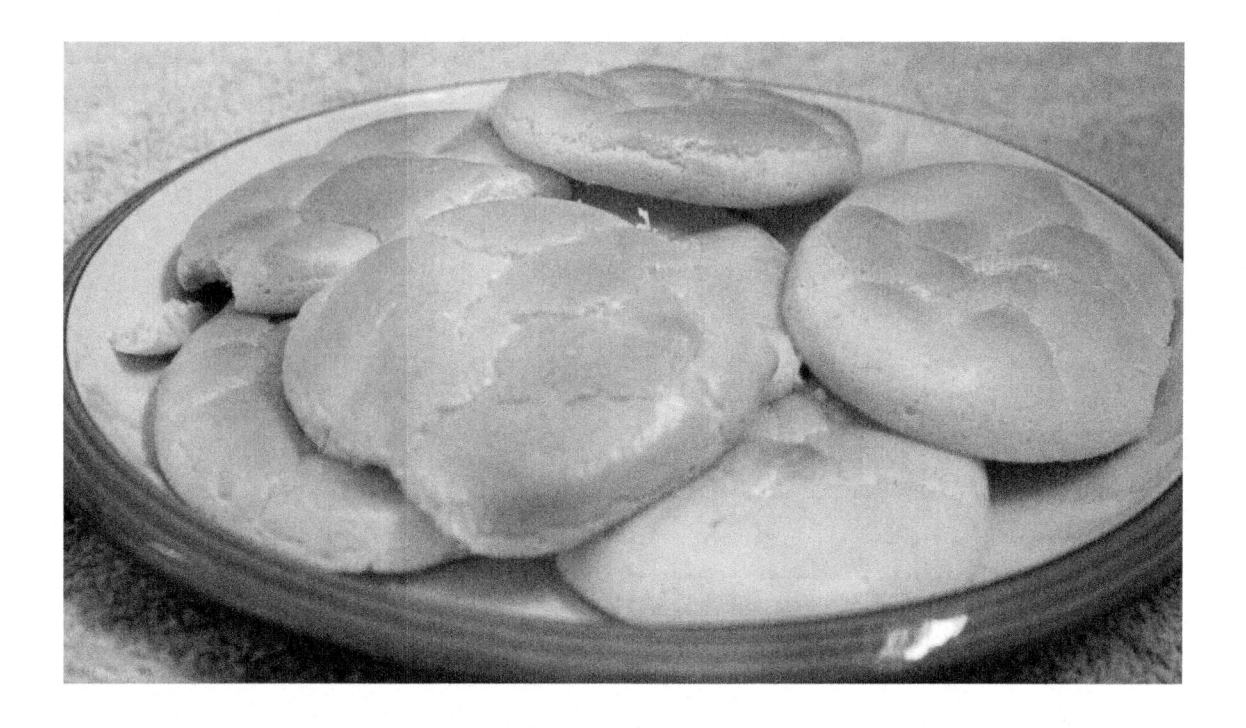

Easy French Toast

Yields: 1 serving (1 slice)

Nutrition Facts: Amount per serving (1 slice)

- Carbohydrates – +2.58g
- Protein – +3.61g
- Total Fat –+12.69g
- Calories – +138

Ingredients:

a. Pick any loaf bread recipe from **Chapter 1: Keto Sweet and Savory Breads** that you prefer. Add the nutrition facts from the base recipe you'll be using
b. 1 tbsp. whole milk
c. 1 tbsp. butter, unsalted, for frying
d. 1 large egg

Directions:

1. Whisk the milk and egg together.
2. Heat the butter over medium-low heat in a non-stick skillet.
3. Dip both sides of your bread into the mixture.

4. Fry each side of the bread for 3-5 minutes. Press on the center of the bread while frying
5. Top any kind of topping you desire.

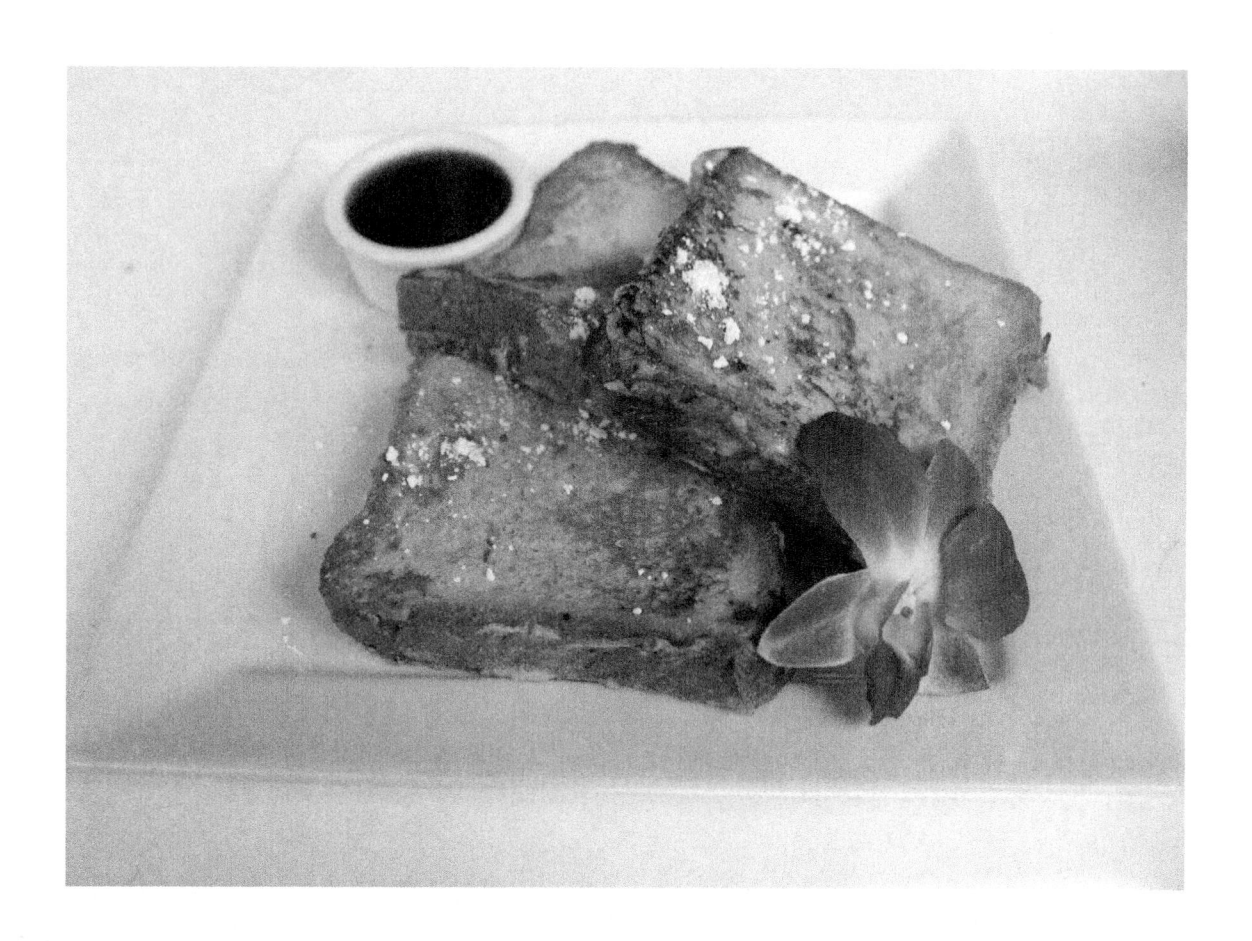

Sandwich Bread

Yields: 1 loaf (10 slices)

Nutrition Facts: Amount per serving (1 slice)

- ➢ Carbohydrates –3.5g
- ➢ Protein – 4.3g
- ➢ Total Fat –12.8g
- ➢ Calories – 255

Ingredients:

a. 2 cups almond flour

b. ½ cup almond milk

c. ¼ cup flaxseed, ground

d. ¼ cup butter, melted

e. 1 tbsp. baking powder

f. ¼ tsp. salt

g. 4 eggs

Directions:

1. Follow the directions for the **Broccoli & Cheddar Breakfast Bread** recipe. But, use these ingredients instead. Also, bake for 30 minutes in 400° F (200° C).

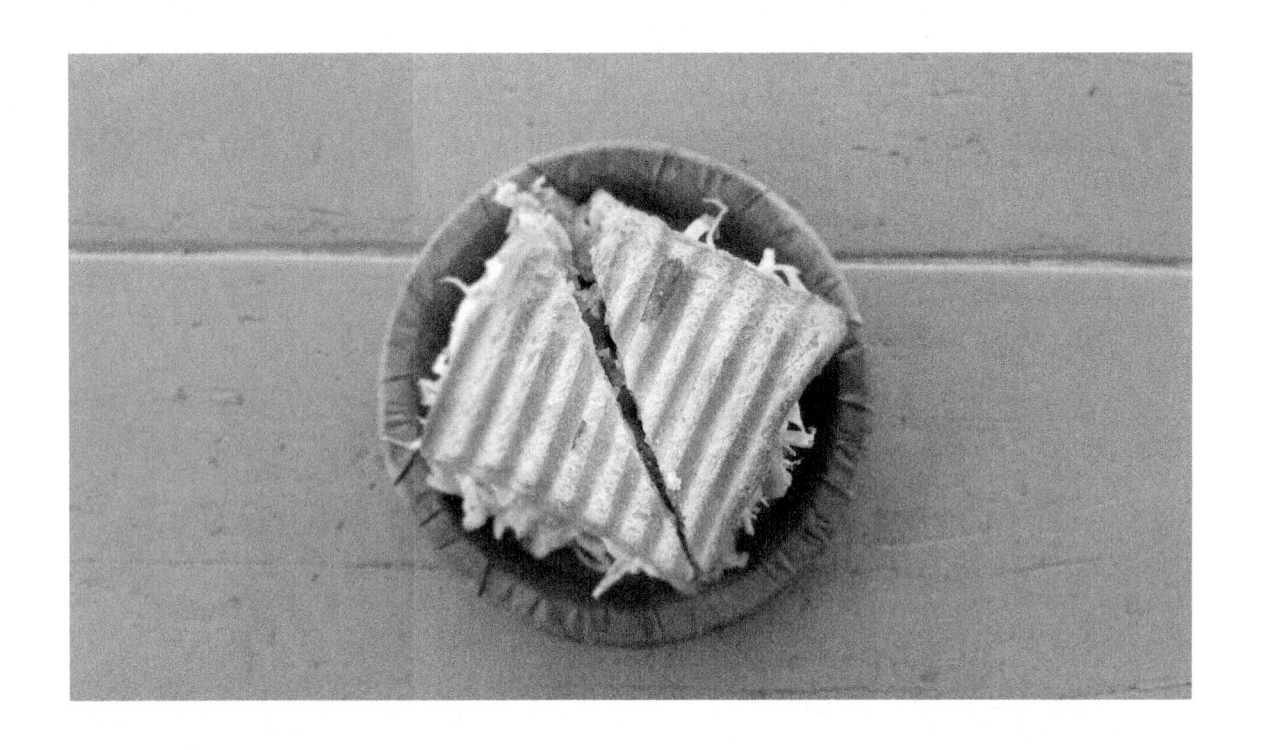

Almond Flour Loaf

Yields: 1 loaf (12 slices)

Nutrition Facts: Amount per serving (1 slice)

- ➢ Carbohydrates –4.1g
- ➢ Protein – 5.7g
- ➢ Total Fat –14.2g
- ➢ Calories – 160

Ingredients:

a. 2 cups almond flour
b. ½ cup + 2 tbsp. warm water
c. ¼ cup butter, melted
d. 2 tbsp. psyllium husk powder
e. 1 ½ tsp. baking powder
f. ½ tsp. xanthan gum
g. A dash of salt
h. 2 eggs + 2 egg whites, left at room temperature

Directions:

1. Preheat the oven to 350° F (180° C). Line a 7x3.5-inch loaf tin with parchment paper.

2. Beat the eggs well. Then, add all the remaining ingredients until you form a dough.
3. Transfer the dough to the loaf tin. Bake for 45 minutes or until the bread passes the toothpick test.

Spinach and Feta Bread

Yields: 1 serving

Nutrition Facts: Amount per serving (1 serving)

- Carbohydrates –4.1g
- Protein – 5.7g
- Total Fat –14.2g
- Calories – 160

Ingredients:

a. 1 tbsp. coconut flour
b. 1 tbsp. almond flour
c. 1 tbsp. butter, melted
d. 1 tbsp. almond milk
e. ¼ tsp. baking powder
f. ¼ cup spinach, finely chopped
g. 1 tbsp. feta, crumbled
h. 1/8 tsp. salt

Directions:

1. Preheat the oven to 400° F (200° C) and prepare a greased ramekin.

2. In a bowl, beat the egg. Then, the rest of the ingredients except for the spinach and feta.

3. Mix in the spinach and feta. Then, transfer the batter into your prepared ramekin.

4. Bake for 10-12 minutes or until done. Remove the bread from the ramekin and serve.

Psyllium Husk & Coconut Flour Loaf

Yields: 1 loaf (15 slices)

Nutrition Facts: Amount per serving (1 slice)

- ➢ Carbohydrates –6g
- ➢ Protein – 3g
- ➢ Total Fat –13.3g
- ➢ Calories – 127

Ingredients:

a. 1 cup coconut flour

b. ¾ cup warm water

c. ½ cup olive oil

d. ¼ cup coconut oil, melted

e. 6 tbsp. psyllium husks, ground finely

f. 1 ½ tsp. baking soda

g. ¾ tsp. sea salt

h. 2 large eggs + 2 cups egg whites

Directions:

1. Preheat the oven to 350° F (180° C). Prepare an 8x4-inch loaf tin lined with parchment paper.
2. Mix all the ingredients together until well-combined.

3. Bake the bread for 45-55 minutes until edges turn brown or until it passes the toothpick test.
4. Let the bread cool for 15 minutes before removing from the loaf tin and slicing.

Flatbread

Yields: 8 pieces

Nutrition Facts: Amount per serving (1 piece)

- Carbohydrates –0.8g
- Protein – 3.6g
- Total Fat –4.5g
- Calories – 56

Ingredients:

a. ¾ cup mozzarella, melted
b. 2 tbsp. almond flour
c. 1 tbsp. cream cheese, melted
d. 1 tbsp. basil
e. 1 tbsp. garlic powder
f. 1 egg

Directions:

1. Preheat your oven to 350° F (180° C) and prepare a greased ramekin.
2. Mix all the ingredients together except for the garlic powder.
3. Divide the mixture into 8 and flatten each portion on a baking sheet. Sprinkle the garlic on top of the bread.

4. Bake for 20 minutes or until edges start to brown.

Buttery Garlic Bread

Yields: 1 loaf (14 slices)

Nutrition Facts: Amount per serving (1 slice)

- ➢ Carbohydrates –5g
- ➢ Protein – 5g
- ➢ Total Fat –14g
- ➢ Calories – 173

Ingredients:

a. 7 oz. full-fat cream cheese, softened
b. 2 garlic cloves, crushed + 1 clove, crushed for the glaze
c. ¼ cup butter, melted for the glaze
d. 1 cup almond flour
e. 3 tbsp. psyllium husks
f. 3 tbsp. coconut flour
g. 1 tsp. salt
h. 6 eggs

Directions:

1. Preheat your oven to 350° F (180° C). Line a baking sheet with parchment paper.

2. Beat the cream cheese and 2 crushed garlic cloves together. Then, add the eggs one at a time while continuing to whisk.
3. Add in the rest of the ingredients and fold gently until you form a dough.
4. Shape the dough into a loaf on the baking sheet. Set aside.
5. Mix the butter and garlic to make the glaze. Brush ¼ of the garlic butter on the dough. Save the rest for later.
6. Bake for 20 minutes. Halfway through baking, score the top of the bread to cook evenly. The bread should turn golden brown once done.
7. Cut the bread into 14 slices and drizzle the rest of the glaze on top before serving.

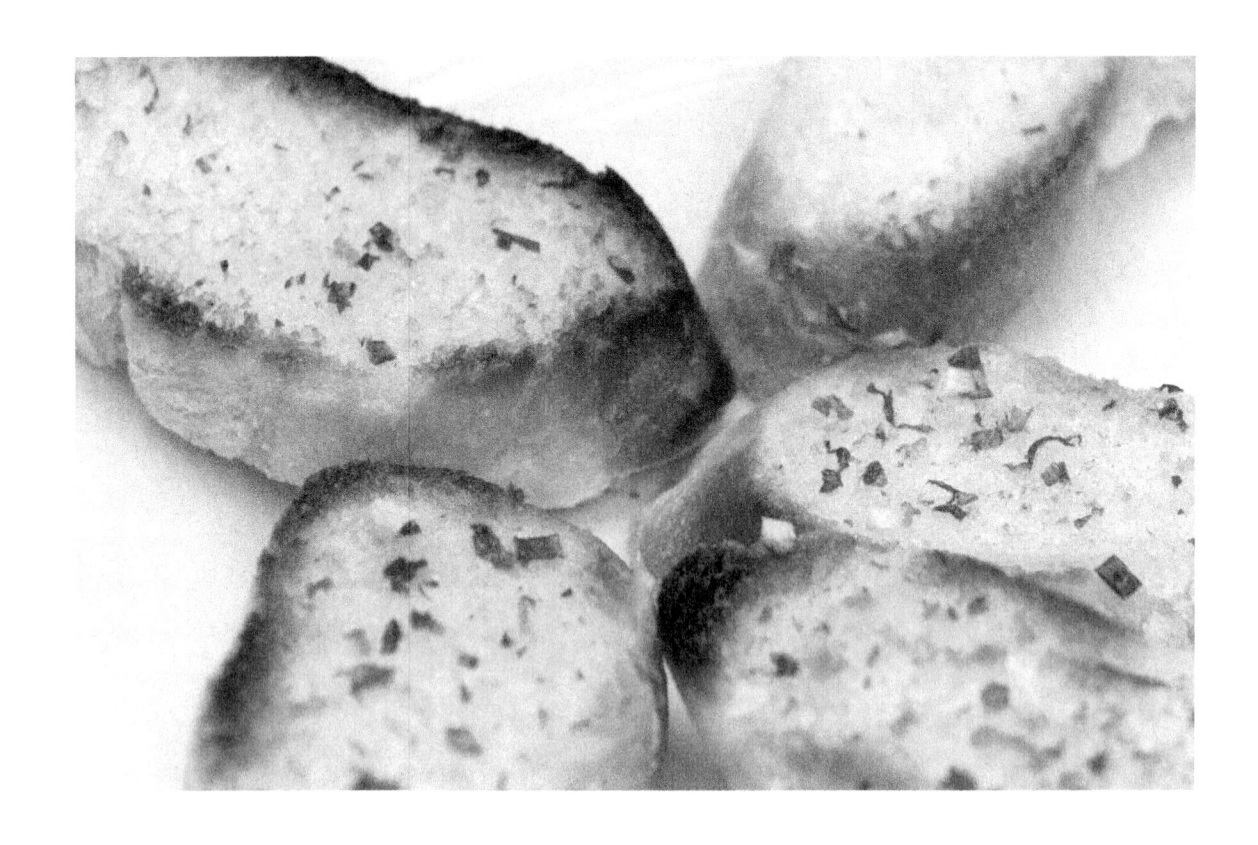

Cheese & Bacon Bread

Yields: 1 loaf (10 slices)

Nutrition Facts: Amount per serving (1 piece)

- Carbohydrates – 0.8g
- Protein – 3.6g
- Total Fat – 4.5g
- Calories – 56

Ingredients:

a. 7 oz. bacon, driced
b. 1 ½ cups almond flour
c. 1 cup cheddar, grated
d. 1/3 cup sour cream
e. 4 tbsp. butter, melted
f. 1 tbsp. baking powder
g. 2 eggs

Directions:

1. Preheat your oven to 300° F (150° C). Grease and line a loaf tin with parchment paper.
2. Cook the bacon in a pan until crispy. Set aside.

3. Mix the baking powder and flour in a bowl. In a separate bowl, whisk the eggs and sour cream until smooth.
4. Add the egg mixture to the flour mixture. Mix until well-combined.
5. Then, mix in the melted butter. Finally, fold the cheese and bacon into the batter.
6. Transfer the batter to the loaf tin. Bake for 45-50 minutes or until the bread passes the toothpick test.
7. Let the bread cool to firm up before slicing.

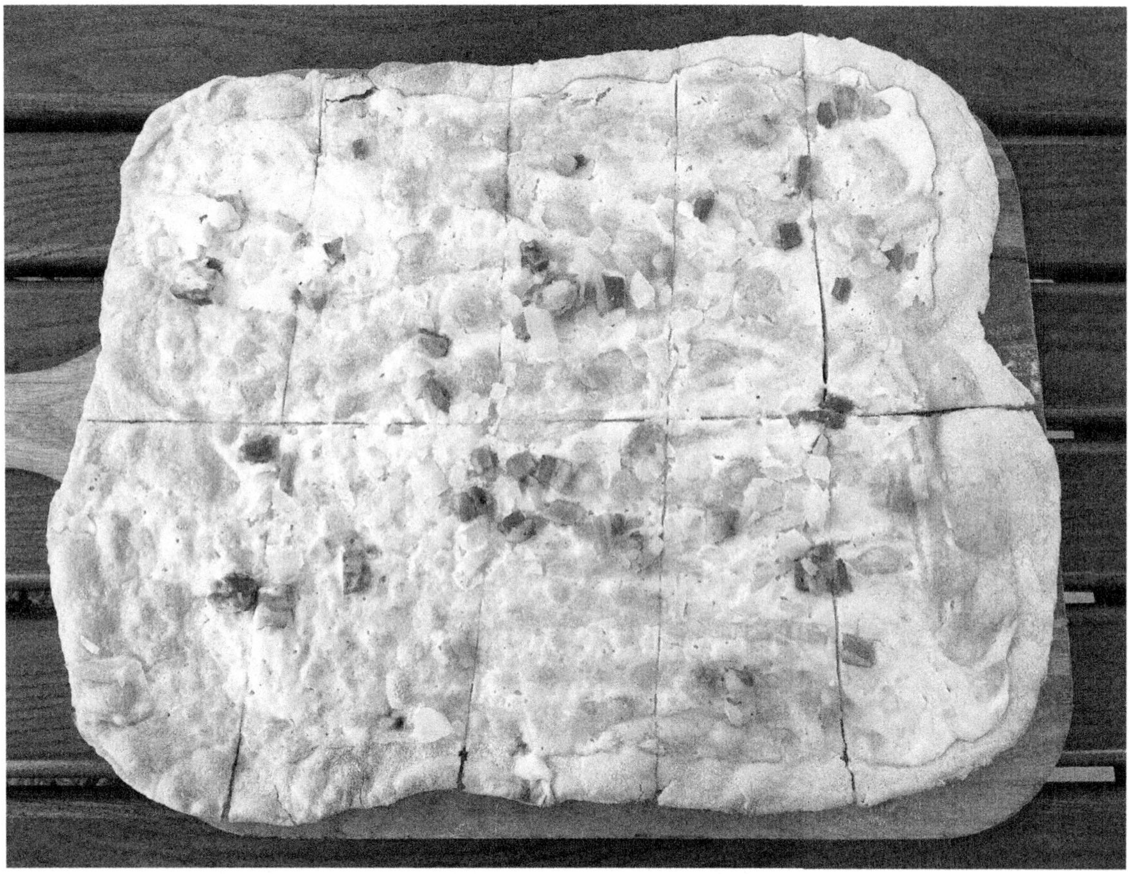

Dinner Rolls

Yields: 9 dinner rolls

Nutrition Facts: Amount per serving (1 dinner roll)

- Carbohydrates – 5g
- Protein – 5g
- Total Fat – 12g
- Calories – 149

Ingredients:

a. 1/3 cup coconut flour
b. ¼ cup almond flour
c. ¼ cup ghee, melted
d. ¼ cup water
e. ¼ cup psyllium husk powder
f. 2 tsp. olive oil
g. 1 tsp. baking soda
h. 1 tsp. baking powder
i. 4 eggs

Directions:

1. Preheat your oven to 350° F (180° C) and prepare a lined baking sheet.

2. Mix all the dry ingredients together until well-combined.
3. In a separate bowl, combine the wet ingredients and mix well.
4. Combine the wet and dry ingredients. Mix well to form a soft dough. Let it rest for about 5 minutes to firm up.
5. Divide the dough into 9 equal portions and form into balls.
6. Place them on the baking sheet and bake for about 25-30 minutes. Reduce the temperature to 300° F (150° C) for the last 10 minutes of baking.

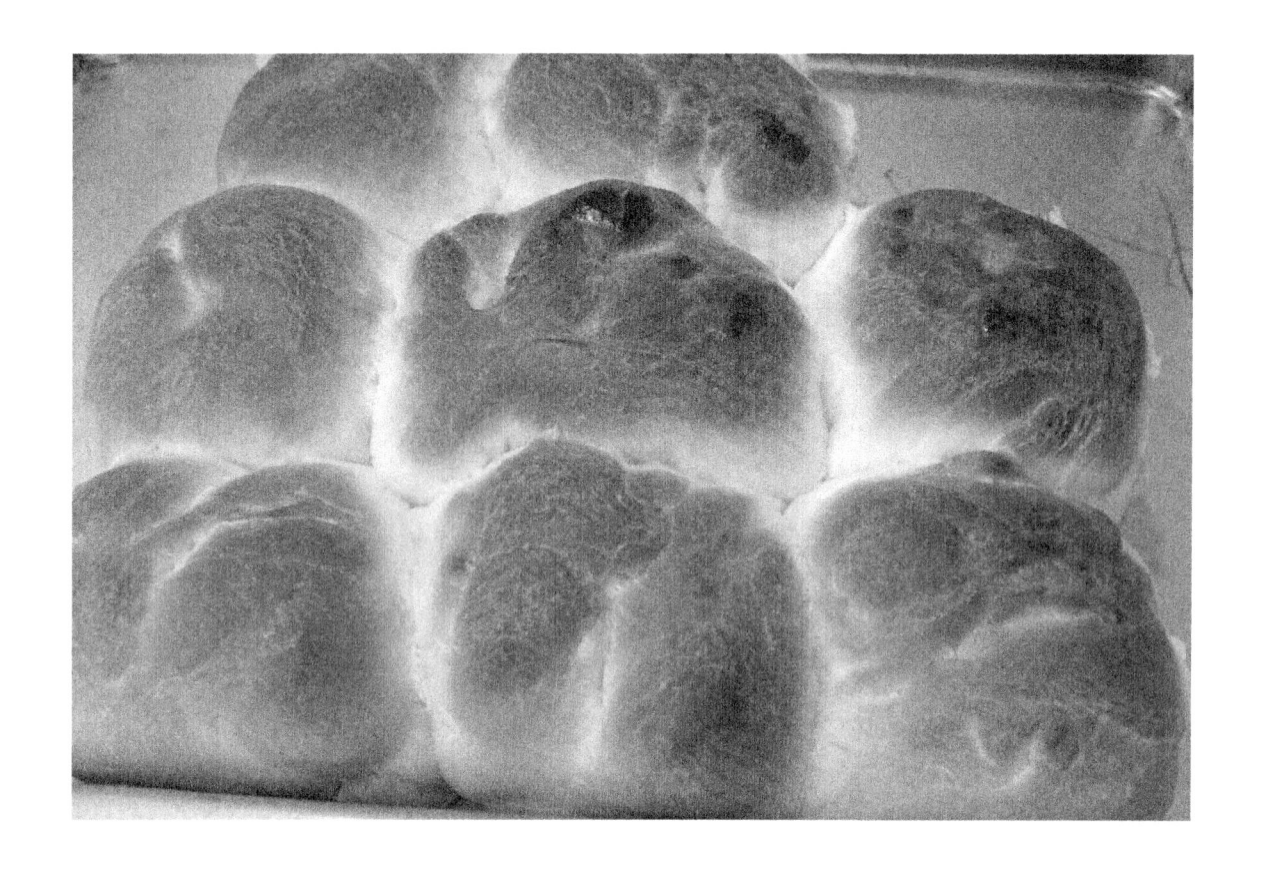

Irish Soda Bread

Yields: 1 loaf (10 slices)

Nutrition Facts: Amount per serving (1 slice)

- ➤ Carbohydrates –0.8g
- ➤ Protein – 3.6g
- ➤ Total Fat –4.5g
- ➤ Calories – 56

Ingredients:

a. 1 oz. raisins
b. 1 ¼ cups almond flour
c. 2 tbsp. coconut flour
d. 2 tbsp. sour cream
e. ½ tbsp. Swerve sweetener
f. ½ tbsp. apple cider vinegar
g. 1 tsp. baking powder
h. 1 tsp. baking soda
i. 1/8 tsp. kosher salt
j. 2 large eggs, whisked

Directions:

1. Preheat your oven to 350° F (180° C). Grease an 8-inch cast iron pan.
2. Add all the dry ingredients and the raisins in a bowl. Mix well to remove any clumps.
3. Then, add the remaining ingredients and mix until well-combined.
4. Place the dough in the greased pan and shape into an oval loaf. Score the top of the bread with an X. Sprinkle with extra Swerve.
5. Bake for about 25-28 minutes or until it becomes golden brown and passes the toothpick test.
6. Completely cool the bread before removing from the pan and slicing.

Microwaveable Hamburger Bun

Yields: 1 bun

Nutrition Facts: Amount per serving (1 bun)

- Carbohydrates – 5g
- Protein – 9g
- Total Fat – 35g
- Calories – 379

Ingredients:

a. 3 tbsp. almond flour

b. 1 ½ tbsp. olive oil

c. ½ tsp. baking powder

d. 1 egg

Directions:

1. Mix the flour and baking powder well to remove clumps. Then, mix in the egg and oil.
2. Beat the mixture well until well-blended. You can use any small microwaveable bowl to cook the bread.
3. Microwave the bread for 90 seconds on high.
4. Cut the hamburger bun and use as you wish.

Naan Bread

Yields: 8 pieces

Nutrition Facts: Amount per serving (1 piece)

- Carbohydrates – 3g
- Protein – 1.3g
- Total Fat – 4.9g
- Calories – 62

Ingredients:

a. 1 cup water, boiling
b. ½ cup coconut flour
c. 2 tbsp. ghee, melted
d. 2 tbsp. whole psyllium husks
e. ¼ tsp. salt
f. ¼ tsp. baking powder
g. 1 egg

Directions:

1. Mix all the ingredients together until you form a dough. Knead, then refrigerate for an hour.
2. Divide the dough into 8 portions. Roll each portion into balls and flatten into desired shape.

3. Cook the bread over medium heat in a cast iron skillet. Cook each side for about 2 minutes or until it starts to become golden brown and puffy.

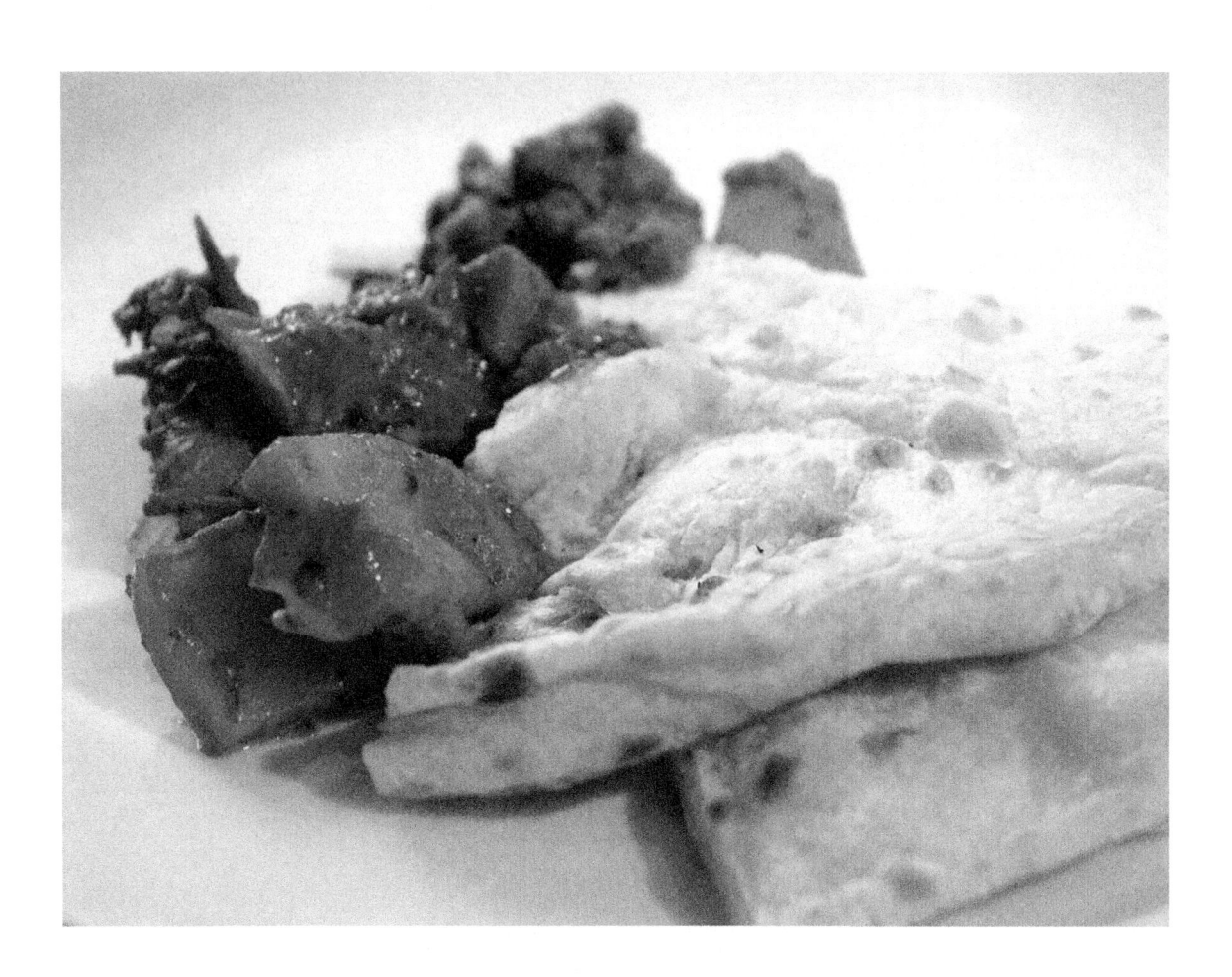

Pumpkin Bread Loaf

Yields: 1 loaf (12 slices)

Nutrition Facts: Amount per serving (1 slice)

- Carbohydrates – 9g
- Protein – 8g
- Total Fat – 18g
- Calories – 215

Ingredients:

a. 2 cups blanched almond flour
b. ¾ cup Erythritol sweetener
c. ¼ cup pumpkin puree
d. ½ cup coconut flour
e. 1/3 cup butter, melted
f. ¼ cup pumpkin seeds
g. 2 tsp. pumpkin spice
h. 2 tsp. baking powder, gluten-free
i. ¼ tsp. sea salt
j. 4 large eggs, beaten

Directions:

1. Preheat your oven to 350° F (180° C). Prepare a 9x5-inch loaf tin lined with parchment paper.
2. Combine the flours, sweetener, pumpkin spice, salt, and baking powder in a bowl. Mix until well-combined.
3. Then, add in the puree, eggs, and butter. Mix everything well.
4. Pour the batter into the loaf tin and smoothen the top. Sprinkle with the seeds and press lightly.
5. Bake for 50 minutes up to an hour or until it passes the toothpick test.
6. Cool it completely before taking out of the pan. Slice into 12 pieces.

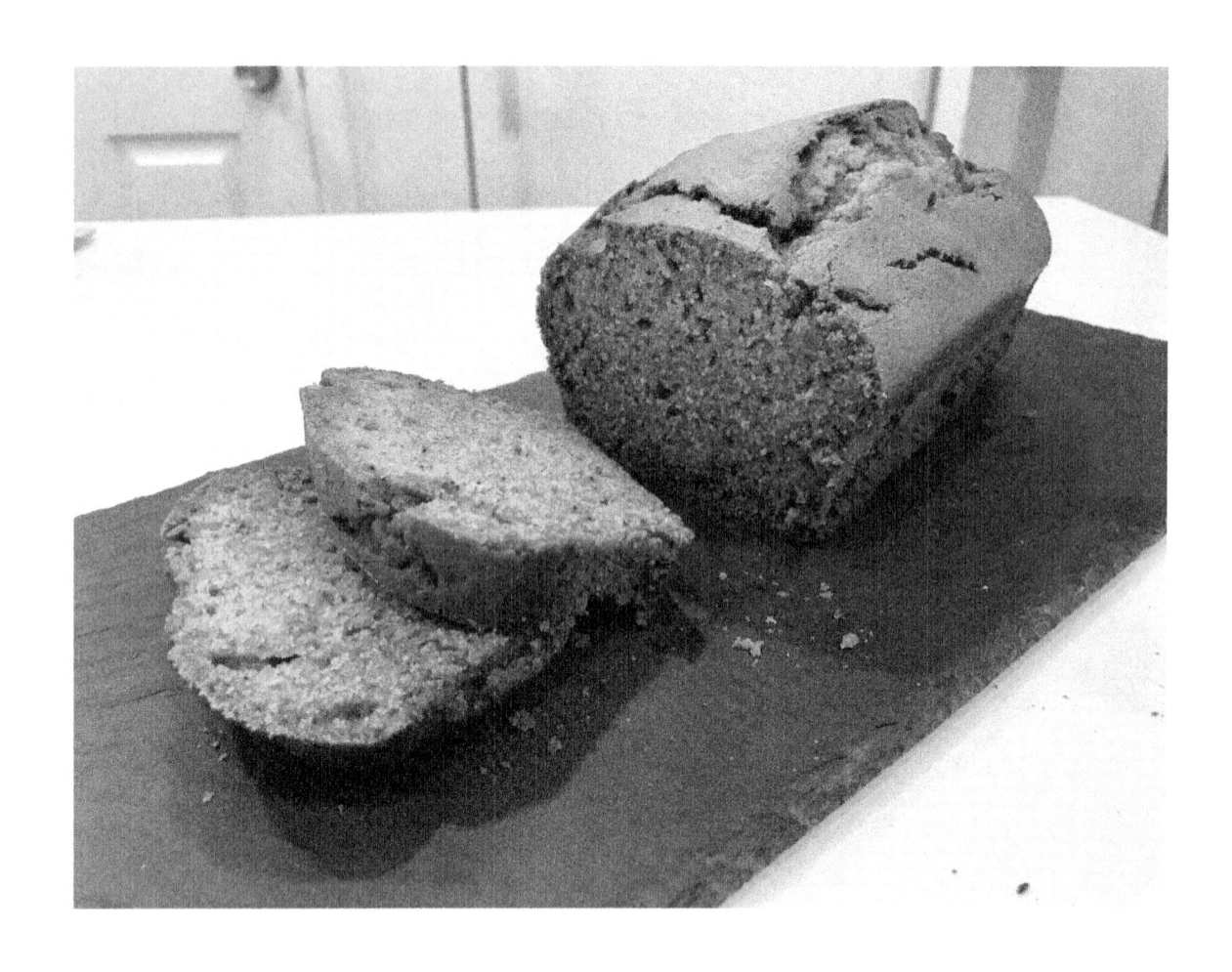

Pork Rind Bread

Yields: 12 slices

Nutrition Facts: Amount per serving (1 slice)

- ➢ Carbohydrates – 1g
- ➢ Protein – 9g
- ➢ Total Fat – 13g
- ➢ Calories – 166

Ingredients:

a. 8 oz. cream cheese
b. 2 cups mozzarella, grated
c. ¼ cup parmesan, grated
d. 1 cup pork rinds, crushed
e. 1 tbsp. baking powder
f. 3 large eggs

Directions:

1. Preheat your oven to 375° F (190° C). Prepare a 12x17-inch baking sheet lined with parchment paper.
2. Melt the mozzarella and cream cheese together and mix well.
3. Add the pork rinds, parmesan, baking powder, and egg. Mix until well-combined.

4. Spread the batter onto the baking sheet.
5. Bake for 15-20 minutes until the top browns lightly.
6. Let it cool for a few minutes before removing from the pan. Slice into 12 pieces equally.

Flaxseed Tortilla Wraps

Yields: 6 tortillas

Nutrition Facts: Amount per serving (1 tortilla)

- Carbohydrates – 2.3g
- Protein – 5.8g
- Total Fat – 6.5g
- Calories – 86

Ingredients:

a. ¼ cup mozzarella, grated
b. 6 tbsp. milled flax seeds
c. 6 tbsp. water
d. ¼ tsp. xanthan gum
e. 3 large eggs

Directions:

1. Mix all the ingredients together using a food processor until well-combined
2. Heat some oil or butter in a pan over medium heat. It's best to use an 8-inch pan.

3. Spoon 2 tbsp. of the batter into the pan. Swirl around to fill the pan. Let the top bubble, then flip the wrap over. Continue to cook until the other side turns brown.

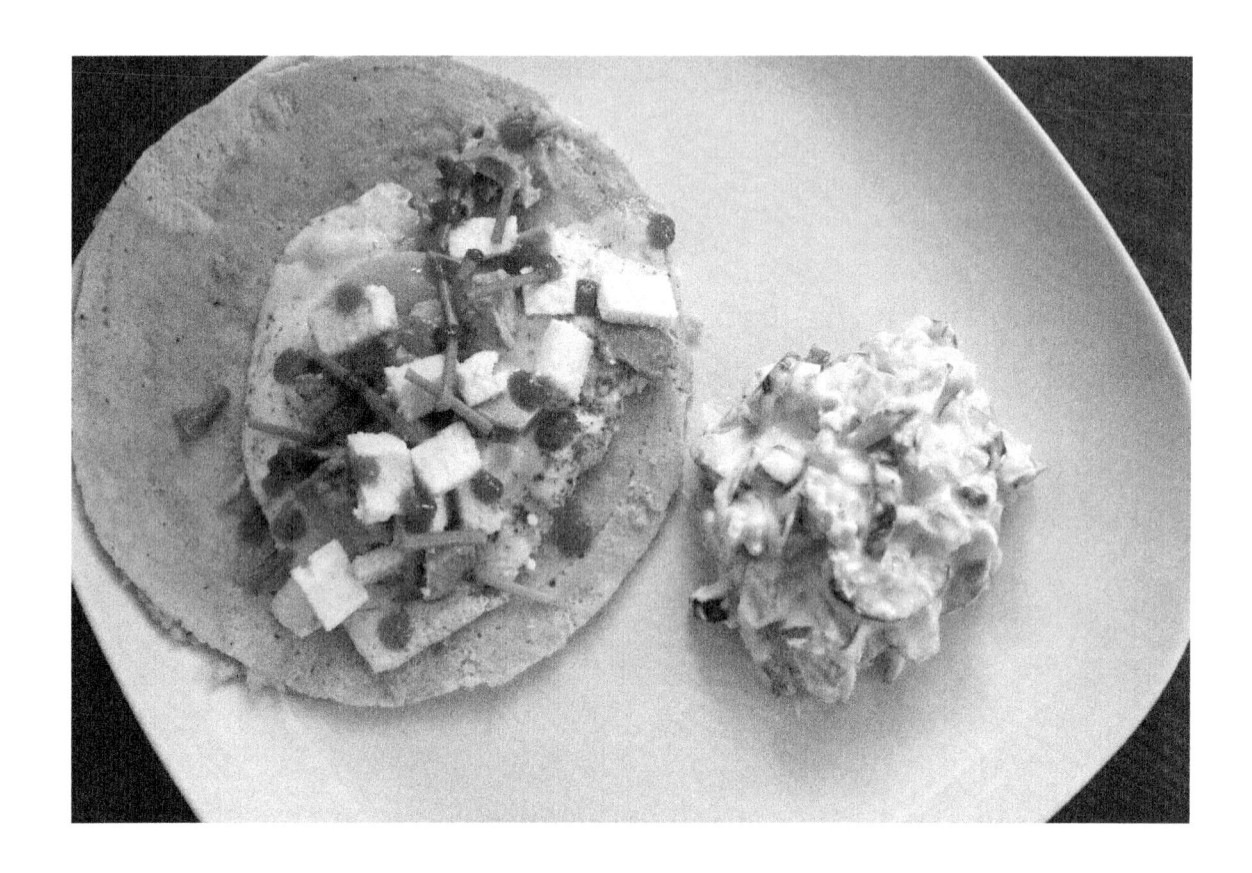

Basic Biscuits

Yields: 8 biscuits

Nutrition Facts: Amount per serving (1 biscuit)

- Carbohydrates – 2g
- Protein – 2g
- Total Fat – 13g
- Calories – 205

Ingredients:

a. 1 ¼ cups almond flour

b. 1/3 cup mozzarella, grated

c. 1/3 cup sour cream

d. 5 tbsp. butter, melted

e. ½ tsp. sea salt

f. ½ tsp. baking powder

g. 2 large eggs

Directions:

1. Preheat your oven to 400° F (200° C). Grease an 8-piece muffin tin with some cooking spray.
2. Mix all the ingredients together until well-combined.

3. Equally distribute the batter into 8 cups of the muffin tin. They should only be 2/3 full.
4. Bake for 10-15 minutes until the tops turn light golden. Let them cool for 3 minutes.

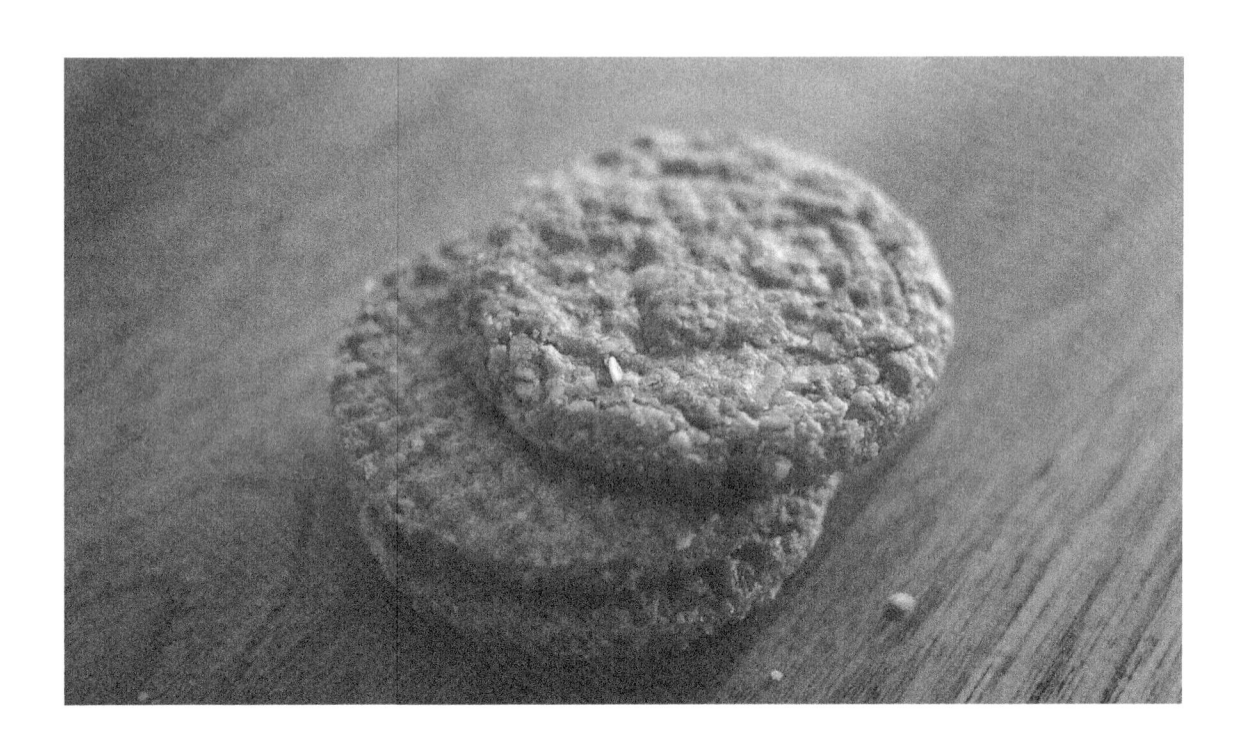

Cheesy Garlic Biscuits

Yields: 14 biscuits

Nutrition Facts: Amount per serving (1 biscuit)

- ➢ Carbohydrates – 4g
- ➢ Protein – 5g
- ➢ Total Fat – 15g
- ➢ Calories – 169

Ingredients:

a. 1 cup blanched almond flour
b. ¾ cup parmesan, grated
c. ½ cup coconut oil, melted
d. 1/3 cup coconut flour
e. 1 tbsp. dried parsley
f. 2 tsp. baking powder, gluten-free
g. 6 garlic cloves, minced
h. 5 large eggs

Directions:

1. Preheat your oven to 350° F (180° C) and prepare a lined baking sheet.

2. Mix all the dry ingredients in a mixing bowl. Then, stir in the wet ingredients. Mix well and let it sit for a few minutes and let it thicken.

3. Place a tablespoonful of the batter onto your baking sheet. Shape it into a biscuit and flatten it lightly. Repeat until you use up all the batter. You should get 14 pieces.

4. Sprinkle extra parmesan on top if you prefer. Then, bake for 15-20 minutes or until the biscuits are golden brown and firm.

Yogurt Herbed Biscuits

Yields: 6 biscuits

Nutrition Facts: Amount per serving (6 biscuits)

- ➢ Carbohydrates – 4g
- ➢ Protein – 5g
- ➢ Total Fat – 10g
- ➢ Calories – 111

Ingredients:

a. 1 cup coconut flour

b. ¼ cup plain yogurt

c. 2 tsp. baking powder

d. 2 tsp. fresh dill

e. 1 tsp. onion powder

f. A pinch of sea salt

g. 1 egg, beaten

Directions:

1. Preheat your oven to 350° F (180° C). Line a baking sheet with parchment paper.
2. Mix all the dry ingredients until well-combined. Then, fold in the egg and yogurt. Mix until you get a frothy and thick batter.

3. Scoop the batter onto the parchment paper dividing it into 6 portions equally.
4. Bake for 15 minutes until it turns golden brown. Let it cool for a bit to firm up.

Basic Almond Biscotti

Yields: 10 pieces of biscotti

Nutrition Facts: Amount per serving (1 piece)

- ➢ Carbohydrates – 0.5g
- ➢ Protein – 4g
- ➢ Total Fat – 5.7g
- ➢ Calories – 70

Ingredients:

a. ¼ cup + 2 tbsp. almond flour

b. ¼ cup almonds, chopped

c. 3 tbsp. butter, melted

d. 2 tsp. Stevia sweetener

e. ½ tsp. baking powder

f. ½ tsp. vanilla extract

g. 1 egg, beaten

Directions:

1. Preheat your oven to 350° F (180° C) and prepare a greased baking sheet.
2. Combine the flour, almonds, and baking powder together.

3. Mix in the butter, vanilla, Stevia, and egg. Continue to stir until you form a firm dough.
4. Create a 1-cm thick log with the dough. Slice the bread into 10 equal sizes.
5. Place the biscotti on the baking sheet and bake for 10 minutes.
6. Then, take the biscuits out of the oven and reduce the oven temperature to 325° F (170° C).
7. Turn the biscotti and bake for an additional 10-15 minutes or until they turn golden brown.

Caramel & Chocolate Biscotti

Yields: 16 pieces of biscotti

Nutrition Facts: Amount per serving (1 piece)

- Carbohydrates – 4g
- Protein – 3g
- Total Fat – 12g
- Calories – 134

Ingredients:

a. 2 ¼ cups almond flour
b. ¼ cup pecans, toasted and chopped
c. ¼ cup Stevia sweetener
d. ¼ cup cold butter, cubed
e. 2 tbsp. chocolate chips, sugar-free
f. 2 tbsp. Erythritol sweetener
g. 2 tbsp. coconut flour
h. 1 tbsp. caramel coffee syrup, sugar-free
i. ¾ tsp. baking powder
j. ½ tsp. xanthan gum
k. 1 egg

Directions:

1. Preheat your oven to 325° F (170° C) and prepare a greased baking sheet.
2. Mix all the ingredients together except for the butter, egg, and syrup. Continue mixing until well-combined.
3. Then, add a few cubes of the butter at a time while mixing. Make sure everything's well-blended before adding the syrup and egg. Mix until you form a dough.
4. Place the dough on a sheet of parchment paper. Then, form it into a loaf that's 2-inch thick and 10-inch long.
5. Transfer to the baking sheet and bake for 20 minutes.
6. Take out from the oven and reduce the oven temperature to 300° F (150° C).
7. Let the loaf cool for 30 minutes before slicing into 16 pieces. Then, place the slices back on the baking sheet with the cut-size down.
8. Bake for an additional 10 minutes. Cool completely before serving.

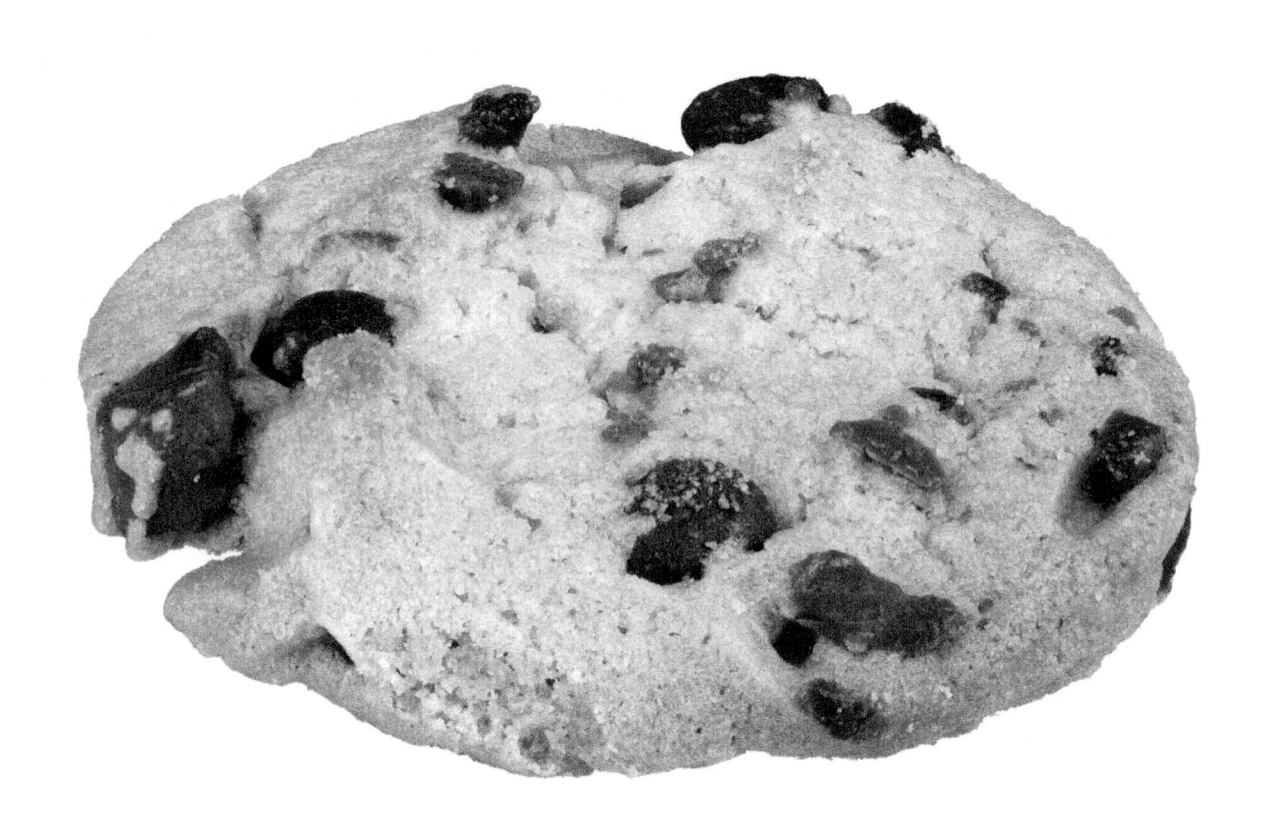

CONCLUSION

I'd like to thank you and congratulate you for transiting my lines from start to finish.

I hope this book was able to help you continue enjoy eating bread while on a ketogenic diet. You can now ask your families and friends who can't say no to bread to start their keto diet.

The next step is to get the right equipment and ingredients you need and start baking!

I wish you the best of luck!

MEAL PREP CHAPTER 2

On Mindful Eating and Curbing Hunger

Switching to a healthier lifestyle, especially after you've been used to doing things a particular way for so long will take some adjustment. There will be challenges and you might find yourself falling behind at certain points—understand that this is totally fine. What matters is that you get back on track, exert a bit more effort, and make some necessary changes that will support the kind of life you want to have.

When it comes to eating healthier, it's more than just selecting the right food and doing portion control. Your overall mental approach matters just as much and being mindful about how you do things can really help make things easier. With that said, here are a few Do's and Don'ts to keep in mind.

The Do's

1. Do start with your shopping list.

Always take your time and make sure you feel focused when writing your list. Mindfulness is key when it comes to creating the right grocery list that will benefit your goals. Think about how you've been feeling lately—what does your body require at the moment? With that in mind, start putting together your choices and edit it as you go.

2. Do savor your meals.

Here's the thing, most people actually rush through their meals because of various reasons. Some may not have a lot of time to spare, whilst there are those who want to use that time for something else "more important". However, it is important to relish your food; take the time to enjoy its flavor, its aroma, and chew properly. Eating mindfully also makes you feel sated for a longer period of time.

3. Do the "mouth full, hands empty" mantra.

This means that you should set your cutlery down in between mouthfuls of food. Quite similar to the previous tip, this is meant to help slow your eating and enable you to better appreciate your food. Not only that, doing this can actually help increase the response of your gut peptides. You'll feel full for longer and keep you from overeating.

4. Always wait a minute or two before going back for seconds.

This allows the food you just ate to settle down and give you enough time to think if you really want more. Most people have a tendency to immediately go for seconds right after eating, especially if the food is something they really like. However, this often leads to them feeling too full and bloated. So, take your time after finishing your plate. Have some water or a sip of tea, then decide if you really need to refill your plate.

5. Do keep your bigger serving bowls of food off the table and out of sight.

This is to serve the previous step's purpose. If you cannot immediately see or reach the food, you won't be able to refill your plate quickly. It also keeps you from craving more just because you keep seeing food. As you may or may not know, just the mere visual of delicious food can make us overeat. If we can see it and smell even while eating, we're bound to grab more servings.

The Don'ts

6. Don't eat while you're distracted by something.

A lot of us fall into the trap of multi-tasking; in this case, eating whilst doing something else. Maybe you do it while you're watching TV, while you're working, or while you're moving from one place to the next. Sure, it feels good to be accomplishing a lot of things at the same time, but did you know that this can be detrimental to your fitness goals? By doing this, you're likelier to overeat or end up snacking again later. This is because your brain isn't fully processing the fact that you're eating.

So next time, give yourself an hour or 30 minutes to eat your meals.

7. Don't drink too much alcohol before you begin eating.

Aside from its calorie content, research has shown that people who drink more before eating are actually more prone to cheating on their diets.

Alcohol is also known to stimulate are appetites, making it harder for us to say no to food we cannot have.

8. Don't eat when you're feeling stressed.

A lot of us have a tendency to "eat our feelings" as a means of relieving stress or any emotional distress we may be experiencing. Whilst this does seem to work, it can also cause us to overeat and feel guilty later on. Instead of turning to food during stressful moments, try mindfulness meditation instead. This will help turn our attention away from what we're craving (usually very indulgent food items) and is also a healthier alternative to stress eating.

9. Don't forego your diet just because you're eating out.

As we've already established, there are ways of still following your diet even when you're out with friends. Remember, people also tend to eat more when they're in social settings or surrounded by friends. Don't stress yourself out when the menu for an event or a restaurant does not fit into your WW freestyle diet. Where you might not be able to be pickier of what you eat, you can always opt for portion sizes.

Eating mindfully is one thing, but the real challenge often happens when you're trying to beat hunger. It can make just about anyone restless and even cranky—everyone's familiar with this. Here are a few do's and don'ts to keep in mind when it comes to curbing your hunger:

The Do's

10. Do your best to always get enough sleep.

Not getting enough sleep actually affects the balance of your hormones related to the appetite. Research shows that people who have had less than 5 hours of sleep experienced an increase in the ghrelin levels in their body. This is the hormone which actually triggers appetite and decreases leptin levels. Leptin is the hormone that signals our brain when we've had enough food.

11. Do a bit of cardio after eating.

Doing this has a positive effect on our satiety hormones, helping promote a longer feeling of satiety. Research also proves that doing moderate-intensity exercises can curb feelings of hunger. It is also an effective form of distraction, keeping you from unintentionally eating or snacking.

When you start feeling the need to snack, try going for a walk instead. After you get back from it, you're bound to feel less inclined to grab a bag of chips or snack on your favorite treats. Note that the brain actually enjoys when we form new habits so do try and focus on making healthier ones, instead of trying to break your current bad habits. You'll eventually replace them when the good habits stick.

12. Do have a hearty breakfast.

Breakfast is important—essential to our day. Having a hearty one provides our body with the ample fuel it needs to give you a head start on the day. People who begin their day with a protein-rich breakfast are less likely to begin craving snacks halfway through their morning. It also keeps you from overeating when lunchtime comes around, effectively preventing body fat gain and enabling you to manage your hunger better.

The Don'ts

13. Don't eat too many fatty foods.

Having too much dietary fat in your daily meals can actually trigger ghrelin, the hunger hormone. Basically, the fattier the food you eat is, the greater your appetite for it would become. Just think back to all the times you've eaten food like French fries, pizzas, steaks, and so on—it's usually really hard to stop, right? This is why.

Another thing to pay attention to is your low-fat food's total energy content. These type of food is likely to contain great amounts of sugar to compensate for any flavor that's lost due to the low-fat content.

14. Don't deprive yourself of your favorite foods.

It's totally okay to enjoy the foods you love, but make sure you do so moderately. Doing so actually helps you deal with cravings better and makes you feel less guilty about having them as well. Banning a food only serves to increase your craving for it so don't be afraid to have your favorites whenever you really feel like them.

Printed in Great Britain
by Amazon